Circle of Care

CIRCLE OF CARE

Clinical Issues
in Jungian Therapy

WARREN STEINBERG

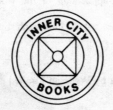

To Catherine, for her love, support and tolerance
To Barry, for his generosity
To Maury, for the friendship
And, of course, to Lea and Jesse, just for being

Canadian Cataloguing in Publication Data

Steinberg, Warren, 1944-
    Circle of care: clinical issues in Jungian therapy

(Studies in Jungian psychology by Jungian analysts; 46)

Includes bibliographical references.

ISBN 0-919123-47-3

1. Transference (Psychology).
2. Countertransference (Psychology).
3. Therapist and patient.   4. Identity (Psychology).
5. Jung, C.G. (Carl Gustav), 1875-1961.
I. Title.   II. Series.

RC489.T73S85 1990   616.89'14   C90-094681-4

INNER CITY BOOKS
Box 1271, Station Q, Toronto, Canada M4T 2P4
Telephone (416) 927-0355

Honorary Patron: Marie-Louise von Franz.
Publisher and General Editor: Daryl Sharp.
Senior Editor: Victoria Cowan.

INNER CITY BOOKS was founded in 1980 to promote the
understanding and practical application of the work of C.G. Jung.

Cover: Band-Bond of Union, 1956, lithograph by M.C. Escher.

Index by Daryl Sharp.

Printed and bound in Canada by Webcom Limited

CONTENTS

See final pages for descriptions of other Inner City Books

Credits

Chapter 1, "Jung's Ideas on Transference," appeared in altered form as "The Evolution of Jung's Ideas on Transference," in *The Journal of Analytical Psychology,* vol. 33, no. 3 (1988).

Portions of chapter 2, "The Therapeutic Utilization of Countertransference," and chapter 3, "The Erotic and Aggressive Countertransferences," appeared in *Quadrant,* vol. 22, no. 1 (1989).

Chapter 4, "The Fear of Therapeutic Progress," was originally presented to the National Conference of Jungian Analysts, San Francisco, October 1989.

Chapter 5, "Idealization: A Clinical Discrimination," appeared originally in altered form in *Quadrant,* vol. 19, no. 2 (1986).

Chapter 6, "Masculine Identity Conflicts," was originally presented as a lecture at the C.G. Jung Foundation, New York, December 1989.

Chapter 7, "Depression," Part I, appeared in altered form as "Depression: A Study of Jung's Ideas," in *The Journal of Analytical Psychology,* vol. 34 (1989); Part II appeared in altered form as "Depression: Some Clinical and Theoretical Observations," in *Quadrant,* vol. 17, no. 1 (1984).

1
Jung's Ideas on Transference

In his major writings on the subject of transference over thirty-four years, Jung's thinking is remarkably consistent. The principal changes in his ideas spring from a continuous deepening and enriching of his initial insights. This is true except for the *value* of the transference, where Jung shows an uncharacteristic tendency to contradict himself.

This chapter presents Jung's ideas on the transference as they developed during his lifetime. Where his initial insight did not evolve significantly, only his original viewpoint will be presented. I will also discuss current misunderstandings about Jung's methods of interpreting the transference and make some speculative comments on the one area in which he is inconsistent.

The Infantile, Reductive Transference

Throughout his writings Jung maintained that the personal, infantile component of neurosis, which manifests in the transference, must first be analyzed reductively. In Jung's earliest published work on transference, he states that the infantile component of the neurotic's personality must be worked through and the prime means of resolution is the analysis of the transference.[1]

In "The Therapeutic Value of Abreaction," Jung asserts that the proper method of analyzing the personal component of the transference is that of reductive analysis.

> The doctor must probe as deeply as possible into the origins of the neurosis in order to lay the foundations of a subsequent synthesis. As a result of reductive analysis, the patient is deprived of his faulty adaptation and led back to his beginnings.[2]

---

[1] "The Theory of Psychoanalysis," *Freud and Psychoanalysis,* CW 4, par. 435. [CW refers throughout to *The Collected Works of C.G. Jung.*]
[2] *The Practice of Psychotherapy,* CW 16, par. 282.

In *Two Essays on Analytical Psychology* Jung added that the resolution of infantile conflicts is primary and takes precedence over the analysis of the collective unconscious.

> As soon as we speak of the collective unconscious we find ourselves in a sphere, and concerned with a problem, which is altogether precluded in the practical analysis of young people or of those who have remained infantile too long. Wherever the father and mother imagos still have to be overcome . . . then we had better make no mention of the collective unconscious . . . . But once the parental transferences and the youthful illusions have been mastered . . . then we must speak of these things.[3]

The way to conquer the infantile relationship to the parents, wrote Jung, is through reductive analysis.

> In the transference all kinds of infantile fantasies are projected. They must be cauterized, i.e., resolved by reductive analysis, and this is generally known as "resolving the transference."[4]

In "The Tavistock Lectures," Jung distinguished between objective and subjective levels of interpretation. On the objective level the patient needs to realize he or she is still looking at the world from the standpoint of a child, "projecting and expecting all the positive and negative authoritative figures of his personal experience."[5]

Finally, in 1946, in "The Psychology of the Transference," his last major article on the subject, Jung reiterated his belief in the necessity of the reductive process:

> Experience has shown that this projection [of past primary relationships] persists with all its original intensity . . . thus creating a bond that corresponds in every respect to the initial infantile relationship, with a tendency to recapitulate all the experiences of childhood on the doctor. In other words, the neurotic maladjustment of the patient is now *transferred* to him. Freud, who was the first to recognize and describe this phenomenon, coined the term "transference neurosis."[6]

---

[3] "On the Psychology of the Unconscious," CW 7, par. 113.

[4] Ibid., par. 96.

[5] *The Symbolic Life*, CW 18, par. 367.

[6] *The Practice of Psychotherapy*, CW 16, par. 357.

In his emphasis on freeing the individual from the parental images through reductive analysis, Jung's attitude is consistent with the ideas expressed by Freud.

Jung's Contribution to the Theory of Transference

Jung differed from Freud in his recognition that the transference and the reductive method had a purposive value. He also pointed out archetypal aspects of the transference, described many of the archetypes projected and formulated technical procedures for the analysis of the archetypal transference. In addition, Jung developed a method of interpretation which he called the synthetic or constructive method. This new method of interpretation did not replace the reductive method, but supplemented it.

The purpose of the transference

Jung perceived that the transference has a purposive value as early as 1913 when he commented that the infantile transference must be resolved since its resolution corresponds with "the urge towards individualization."[7] In the same letter, Jung criticized the purely causal viewpoint and related the transference to psychological imperatives similar to those that lead a bird to build its nest.[8]

In "The Transcendent Function," written in 1916, Jung made his first attempt at formulating a synthetic view of the psychic process in analytical treatment. By the transcendent function Jung meant the patient's unconscious attempt to arrive at a new attitude through the union of conscious and unconscious. The transference mediates the transcendent function when unconscious contents, which are compensatory to a one-sided conscious attitude, are projected onto the analyst. Thus, Jung concluded, transference fantasies are not to be understood merely "in a concretistic-reductive sense, but rather in a constructive one."[9]

By 1921, Jung's ideas about neurosis and the transference were

---

[7] "Some Crucial Points in Psychoanalysis (Jung-Loÿ Correspondence)," *Freud and Psychoanalysis,* CW 4, par. 658.

[8] Ibid., par. 665.

[9] *The Structure and Dynamics of the Psyche,* CW 8, par. 146.

becoming more teleologically oriented. He wrote: "Not only must the patient be able to see the cause and origin of his neurosis, he must also see the legitimate psychological goal towards which he is striving."[10] The transference contains "a creative element, the purpose of which is to shape a way out of the neurosis."[11]

In *Two Essays on Analytical Psychology,* Jung continued to expand the idea that neurosis itself is purposeful, its aim being to create a new balance for the personality by making unconscious contents conscious. He added the view that the patient transfers onto the analyst the specific elements required for the development of the personality, and not just past memories.[12] For example, in "The Tavistock Lectures," Jung reported the following dream from a new patient:

> She was coming to the Swiss frontier. It was day and she saw the custom-house. She crossed the frontier and she went into the custom-house, and there stood a Swiss customs official. A woman went in front of her and he let that woman pass, and then her turn came. She had only a small bag with her, and she thought she would pass unnoticed. But the official looked at her and said: "What have you got in your bag?" She said: "Oh, nothing at all," and opened it. He put his hand in and pulled out something that grew bigger and bigger, until it was two complete beds.[13]

Jung understood that he was the Swiss customs official in the dream and that one of the purposes of the transference was to help the patient resolve her conflicts about marriage, which were symbolized by the two beds.

Therapeutically, it is important to integrate not only the objective value of the projected contents but also their subjective and prospective value. In "The Tavistock Lectures," Jung pointed out that a particular patient needed to understand not only how his mother and father treated him negatively, but also how he repeated that behavior toward himself and others.[14]

---

[10] "The Therapeutic Value of Abreaction," *The Practice of Psychotherapy,* CW 16, par. 293.

[11] Ibid., par. 277.

[12] "On the Psychology of the Unconscious," CW 7, pars. 141-147.

[13] *The Symbolic Life,* CW 18, par. 348.

[14] Ibid., par. 367.

Finally, in 1946, Jung concluded that the fantasy contents which appear in the transference can be understood either reductively or symbolically—as the spiritual meaning of the instincts.[15]

Together with his purposive approach to the transference, Jung developed the related ideas of compensation, empathy and relationship.

Compensation

Compensation is the mechanism through which the psyche automatically regulates itself. If, due to resistances or excessive repressions, ego-consciousness becomes too one-sided, a neurosis develops. The information which compensates the conscious attitude emerges through specific symptoms. The transference, like the neurosis, is an attempt at self-cure, the psychic system striving for balance.

In "The Tavistock Lectures," Jung gave an example of "over-compensation" in the case of a female patient who was extremely intellectual and whose defenses insulated her from relationship. The patient developed an intense erotic transference to Jung. In his understanding, her unconscious arranged this so as to help her develop her inferior, unrelated feeling side.[16]

Compensation can also work to inform the analyst about an unhelpful countertransference. During his work with one woman, Jung dreamed:

> I was walking along a country road through a valley lit by the evening sun. To my right, standing on a steep hill, was a castle, and on the topmost tower, on a kind of balustrade, sat a woman. In order to see her properly I had to bend my head back so far that I got a crick in the neck. Even in my dream I recognized the woman as my patient.[17]

This dream helped Jung realize that he had become frustrated with the woman owing to her resistance. His defensive countertransfer-

---

[15] "The Psychology of the Transference," *The Practice of Psychotherapy*, CW 16, par. 362.

[16] *The Symbolic Life*, CW 18, pars. 338-344.

[17] "On the Psychology of the Unconscious," *The Essays on Analytical Psychology*, CW 7, par. 189.

ence reaction was to devalue his patient. The dream compensated this by having Jung look up to her.

Empathy

Another purposive component of the transference that Jung emphasized is empathy. The patient tries to feel into the personality of the analyst and get into harmony with it, to obtain a good relationship with the analyst by comparing it to earlier relationships. The purpose of this is adaptation. The patient assumes the analyst has the proper attitude toward life and that identifying with the analyst will lead to resolution of the patient's conflicts.[18]

We can assume that a clinician as astute as Jung did not advocate the patient identifying with fantasies of how the analyst would solve a specific problem. Jung undoubtedly meant that there is validity to the patient's attempt to heal through empathy, provided the patient identifies with the analytic attitude, that is, with the analyst's intention to make the unconscious conscious. In this sense one might consider Jung's idea of the healing function of empathy as an early formulation of the concept of introjective identification. Of course, this attempt at adaptation can go awry if the therapist has a defensive attitude toward the unconscious.

Relationship

Jung recognized that it is a characteristic of the neurotic to find it difficult to establish healthy human relationships. One purposive aspect of the transference is the patient's unconscious attempt to do this. Of course, this is doomed to failure because the patient quickly assimilates the analyst to the pathological family situation. The projections cause the analyst to become father, mother or other significant figures and the infantile relationships are resurrected. However, the analyst is also outside the family environment and can, therefore, provide a bridge out of these dynamics.

As the infantile projections are withdrawn the need for healthy relationship becomes clearer. The patient will then turn to the analyst as

---

[18] "Some Crucial Points in Psychoanalysis (Jung-Loÿ Correspondence)," *Freud and Psychoanalysis,* CW 4, pars. 657-662.

an object of purely human relationship in which each individual is guaranteed a place. Writes Jung:

> Naturally this is impossible until all the projections have been consciously recognised; consequently they must be subjected to a reductive analysis before all else, provided of course that the legitimacy and importance of the underlying claim to personal relationship is constantly borne in mind.[19]

Jung returned to the idea of the importance of relationship in the transference in "The Psychology of the Transference," in which he suggested that relationship is a condition for individuation. The ego needs another person on whom to project unconscious contents so that conscious union can then take place.

> The unrelated human being lacks wholeness, for he can achieve wholeness only through the soul, and the soul cannot exist without its other side, which is always found in a "You."[20]

The archetypal transference

At an early stage Jung raised the question of what happened to the energy freed when transference projections are withdrawn from the analyst and resolved. He felt that this energy could not be sublimated by conscious choice and warned against the therapist trying to direct it by suggestion and advice. The energy had its own gradient, Jung said, and would find the application for which it was most suited.

At first, Jung assumed this application would be to some external adaptation. He believed that for most patients, especially those not yet middle-aged, the main cause of neurosis was an avoidance of an external adaptation to life. The disposable energy freed by reductive analysis would gravitate to an object or task in the outer world.

In *Two Essays on Analytical Psychology* Jung introduced the idea of the archetypal transference. He had discovered that, in some unusual cases, after reductive analysis the freed libido does not lead to new external adaptations but follows its own gradient to the collective unconscious and activates archetypes which are then projected in

---

[19] "The Therapeutic Value of Abreaction," *The Practice of Psychotherapy,* CW 16, par. 286.

[20] *The Practice of Psychotherapy,* CW 16, par. 454.

the transference. The ideas he then formulated can be differentiated into two related hypotheses. First, the transference is archetypal, in that collective contents are projected onto the analyst; and second, a purposive development toward individuation is inherent in the transference, that is, the transference process is itself archetypal.

Jung convincingly cited a number of clinical cases to support his first hypothesis. His idea that the transference had a purposive direction, however, rested tenuously on one countertransference-marred example of a woman with a strong positive father complex. She idealized Jung and in her dreams he was inflated into a godlike father figure carrying her like a child. Jung presented the following dream from this patient:

> Her father (who in reality was of small stature) was standing with her on a hill that was covered with wheat-fields. She was quite tiny beside him, and he seemed to her like a giant. He lifted her up from the ground and held her in his arms like a little child. The wind swept over the wheat-fields, and as the wheat swayed in the wind, he rocked her in his arms.[21]

Jung wondered why, in view of the analytic work, her unconscious was holding steadfastly to the idea that he was godlike. The tie was being strengthened rather than attenuated. He concluded

> that the unconscious was trying to *create* a god out of the person of the doctor, as it were to free a vision of God from the veils of the personal, so that the transference to the person of the doctor was no more than a misunderstanding on the part of the conscious mind, a stupid trick played by "sound common sense"? . . . Could the longing for a god be . . . . the highest and truest meaning of that inappropriate love we call "transference"?[22]

It is questionable whether Jung's idea that the individuation process is inherent in the transference is supported by this example. In arriving at his conclusions Jung did not take into account the fact that the patient had run out of money and he implied that he was seeing her without charging a fee.[23] This was undoubtedly a stimulus for

---

21 "The Relations Between the Ego and the Unconscious," CW 7, par. 211.

22 Ibid., par. 214.

23 Ibid., par. 209.

the patient's exaggerated transference fantasy. The idealizing transference could not be diminished because Jung kept on reinforcing it by treating the patient as if she were a child.

The most that can be concluded about the archetypal transference from the examples cited in *Two Essays on Analytical Psychology,* therefore, is that archetypal images appear both spontaneously and reactively. Rather than providing evidence for the idea that the unconscious autonomously tries to individuate through the transference, it could be argued that Jung provided support for the hypothesis that the unconscious presents a corrective to the analyst's countertransference via archetypal imagery.

In his later writings, Jung presented additional material to substantiate the idea that the individuation process underlies the transference. In "The Tavistock Lectures" he compared the transference to initiatory experiences and contended that both serve the same function of detaching energy from the parental images so that it can be transferred to the next phase of development. In this sense the analysand, like the hero, is twice born, once of the natural parents, then, through the transference, the individual experiences a spiritual rebirth and is released from attachment to the parental images.[24]

The idea of the transference as a second birth is also dealt with in "The Psychology of the Transference," where Jung emphasized its developmental purpose.[25] Here Jung again presented the thesis that the transference is a directional archetypal process whose purpose is individuation. Through an analysis of the *Rosarium philosophorum* pictures, Jung showed the parallels between the alchemical and transference processes. He convincingly concluded that just as the real meaning of the alchemical opus, the search for the *lapis,* is a projection of the instinct for wholeness, so the underlying drive in the transference process is the need for inner unity.

The synthetic method

In "The Tavistock Lectures" Jung introduced a general technical plan for analyzing the archetypal transference. The analyst must first help

---

24 *The Symbolic Life,* CW 18, pars. 363-366.
25 *The Practice of Psychotherapy,* CW 16, pars. 455ff.

the patient discriminate the personal from the impersonal contents projected in the transference. Then the impersonal images need to be withdrawn from the analyst so that the personal relationship can be clearly differentiated.

However, unlike the personal transference which is resolved through the reductive analysis of the projections, the archetypal images cannot be dissolved because they belong to the structural elements of the psyche. Hence it is the act of projection itself that must be dissolved. The impersonal images that fall back into the patient must be differentiated from the ego via the method of "objectivation."[26] Jung was here referring to the synthetic method.

The synthetic method has two components: amplification of the symbol and the subjective level of interpretation.

Causal and reductive procedures break down when images from the collective unconscious appear. This kind of material becomes meaningless when reduced to anything personal, but displays meaning if reinforced and amplified. The archetypal image is understood as a symbol which anticipates future developments in the analysand. The synthetic method attempts to comprehend the purpose of the symbol by developing its meanings through parallels supplied by both analyst and patient.

"This procedure widens and enriches the initial symbol," writes Jung, "Certain lines of psychological development then stand out that are at once individual and collective."[27]

Amplification and active imagination are two examples of the synthetic method.

The second component is the subjective level of interpretation. The unconscious product projected onto the analyst, as well as the associations to that product, are regarded not as aspects of the object but as tendencies or characteristics of the analysand. The subjective level of interpretation can be applied to personal as well as archetypal material. Again, the assumption is that it is a purposive process. The unconscious material is projected onto the analyst at this time because it is necessary for the patient to integrate it.

---

[26] *The Symbolic Life,* CW 18, par. 377.
[27] "The Relations Between the Ego and the Unconscious," *Two Essays on Analytical Psychology,* CW 7, par. 493.

The value of the transference.

There is a consistency and evolution to Freud's viewpoint of the transference. He initially experienced the transference as an obstacle to treatment, that is, a resistance. As an inevitable feature of analytic work it was unavoidable, and the analyst had to learn to work with it. As he continued his explorations, Freud recognized that transference was also of great therapeutic value. It provided an opportunity for the patient to repeat in a safe environment the pathological experiences that formed the basis of his or her conflicts. In this new environment these earlier experiences could be shown to be the unconscious motivations for the person's current maladaptive behavior. Transference became the battlefield on which the war of the neurosis could be fought.

There is no such consistency or development in Jung's views on the value of the transference. Quite the contrary, this is the only area in all his writings on transference where Jung continuously contradicts himself. He even contradicts himself in the same article. This is perhaps indicative of some personal emotional conflict that Jung experienced in relation to the issue of transference.

In 1912, Jung declared the discovery of transference to be of "fundamental importance."[28] It served the useful purpose of helping the patient build a bridge from the family relationship to the world outside the family.

In a 1913 letter to Dr. Loÿ, Jung states: "We do not work *with* the 'transference to the analyst,' but *against it and in spite of it.*"[29] This echoes the position initially adopted by Freud (in 1895), seeing the transference solely as an obstacle to treatment.

In 1921, Jung returned to the idea that transference is important and has a positive value when he declared that "the transference is the alpha and omega of psychoanalysis."[30] He again attributed much positive value to the relational benefits he felt the patient derived from

---

28 "The Theory of Psychoanalysis," *Freud and Psychoanalysis,* CW 4, par. 428.

29 "Some Crucial Points in Psychoanalysis (Jung-Loÿ Correspondence)," *Freud and Psychoanalysis,* CW 4, par. 601 (italics in original).

30 "The Therapeutic Value of Abreaction," *The Practice of Psychotherapy,* CW 16, par. 276.

the transference. He also took up a position similar to Freud's by claiming that the transference was "an inevitable feature of every thorough analysis."[31]

In 1926, Jung contradicted the idea of the inevitability of the transference when he said that it was not "a regular phenomenon indispensable to the success of the treatment. Transference is projection, and projection is either there or not there. But it is not *necessary*. . . . The absence of projections to the doctor may in fact considerably facilitate the treatment."[32]

In 1935, Jung returned to his standpoint of 1913 with extreme statements such as:

A transference is always a hindrance; it is never an advantage. You cure in spite of the transference, not because of it.[33]

It is abnormal to have a transference. Normal people never have transferences.[34]

Transference or no transference, that has nothing to do with the cure. . . . If there is no transference, so much the better. You get the material just the same. It is not transference that enables the patient to bring out his material; you get all the material you could wish for from dreams.[35]

Again Jung seemed to favor Freud's original resistance/obstacle model. At other times, however, he recognized that transference, like projection, of which it is an instance, is a normal phenomenon and is merely a way for activated contents to become conscious.[36]

Finally, in 1946, he returned to the inevitability and importance of the transference in analytic treatment.

It is probably no exaggeration to say that almost all cases requiring lengthy treatment gravitate around the phenomenon of transference,

---

[31] Ibid., par. 283.

[32] "On the Psychology of the Unconscious," *The Essays on Analytical Psychology,* CW 7, par. 94, note 13.

[33] "The Tavistock Lectures," *The Symbolic Life,* CW 18, par. 349.

[34] Ibid., par. 350.

[35] Ibid., par. 351.

[36] "The Psychology of the Transference," *The Practice of Psychotherapy,* CW 16, par. 420.

and that the success or failure of the treatment appears to be bound up with it in a very fundamental way. Psychology, therefore, cannot very well overlook or avoid this problem, nor should the psychotherapist pretend that the so-called "resolution of the transference" is just a matter of course.[37]

Medical treatment of the transference gives the patient a priceless opportunity to withdraw his projections, to make good his losses, and to integrate his personality.[38]

Jung now stated his personal preference to not have to work with the transference, especially an intense one, but to work instead with dreams:

I personally am always glad when there is only a mild transference or when it is practically unnoticeable. Far less claim is then made upon one as a person, and one can be satisfied with other therapeutically effective factors.[39]

Discussion

Synthetic and reductive interpretations

There are a number of benefits and dangers to the synthetic approach with regard to the transference. One is that its too ready application prevents unconscious fantasies from having adequate time to manifest in the transference. The patient needs the analyst as a transference object, but if the emerging projection makes the analyst uncomfortable, the analyst may quickly put it back onto the patient. The subjective interpretation then becomes a defense against the patient's frightening unconscious material. This is especially the case when the negative transference begins to emerge or the patient projects sexual wishes onto the analyst.

In addition, the patient's associations to the object may be accurate perceptions rather than distortions. If the analyst is unwilling to acknowledge the patient's valid unconscious perceptions, the subjective level of interpretation provides a ready defense. Similarly, the

---

37 Ibid., p. 164.
38 Ibid., par. 420.
39 Ibid., par. 359.

amplificatory aspect of the synthetic method can be used defensively to collude with the patient in order to avoid mutually frightening personal material that needs to manifest in the transference.

Conversely, on the objective level of interpretation, a danger is that the analyst, the object of the patient's fantasies, will identify with, and attempt to retain, the patient's projections. This danger is especially acute with archetypal transferences and those of a positive nature. For example, an analyst with unresolved narcissistic problems may readily interpret the patient's idealization on the objective level. An analyst with a savior complex will easily identify with the projection of the savior archetype, a common transference projection. One protection against this is the synthetic technique of amplifying the patient's image. The parallels help both the analyst and the patient recognize the impersonal nature of the transferred material.

That Jung recognized these dangers is evident from his emphasis on both the synthetic method and the importance of the object in transference analysis. As a matter of fact, relationship to the object is a requirement of successful individuation, not only because as human beings we need social interaction in order to develop, but because the object is necessary for projection. We get to know ourselves through projection; thus we need to be in a relationship for the unconscious fantasies to become manifest.[40]

There is an erroneous tendency to identify Jungian psychotherapy with the synthetic technique and to speak pejoratively of the reductive method. The latter is considered a Freudian, causal, personalistic approach that fails to satisfy the progressive needs of the personality. The synthetic method, since it was originated by Jung, is quite naturally considered more Jungian. The decision about which technical approach to use ceases to be a clinical decision and becomes a criterion for who is and is not a Jungian analyst. Clinical decisions are then decided on the basis of adherence to theoretical dogma rather than the individual needs of the patient.

Often the antagonism toward the reductive technique is defensively motivated, rooted in the analyst's feelings of inadequacy. During training, the analyst may have become comfortable and com-

---

[40] Ibid., par. 454.

petent with the synthetic approach, but feel insecure when using reductive techniques.

In fact, conflicts about the choice of method have little to do with Jung's actual standpoint. Jung clearly favored choosing an analytic approach based on clinical circumstances.

> Thus we apply a largely reductive point of view in all cases where it is a question of illusions, fictions, and exaggerated attitudes. On the other hand, a constructive point of view must be considered for all cases where the conscious attitude is more or less normal, but capable of greater development . . . or where unconscious tendencies . . . are being misunderstood . . . . Which point of view he shall decide to adopt in any given case must be left to the insight and experience of the analyst.[41]

The tendency to create a dichotomy between the reductive and the synthetic is a serious error and indicates a failure to understand Jung's viewpoint. What underlies this failure, I believe, is a deeper misunderstanding about the causal and purposive points of view.

The synthetic method is associated with a purposive approach to the psyche which takes account of and fosters the goal-oriented needs of the personality. The reductive approach is associated with infantile causality. However, Jung distinguished two kinds of causality: *causa efficiens* and *causa finalis*.[42] *Causa efficiens* refers to the immediately effecting cause and answers the question "Why did it happen?" *Causa finalis* refers to the final cause and answers the question "To what purpose did it happen?"

Reduction to infantile causality is mistakenly understood by some to mean reduction to a *causa efficiens*, an unsatisfactory psychological explanation for those with a purposive point of view. For Jung, however, reduction to infantile causality was a reduction to a *causa finalis*. According to the concept of finality, causes are understood to be means to an end. Reduction to infantile causality is a necessary step in the process of discovering meaning, although it leaves unanswered the question of purpose.

---

[41] "Analytical Psychology and Education," *The Development of Personality,* CW 17, par. 195.
[42] "On the Nature of Dreams," *The Structure and Dynamics of the Psyche,* CW 8, par. 530.

For individuation to occur, the individual often has first to resolve infantile conflicts. The compensatory material needed for the resolution of the psychological disturbance and for further growth of the personality may reside in childhood relationships and conflicts. But if this material is to become conscious a regression is necessary. Regression is experienced through projection onto the analyst, that is, in the transference. Reduction to the infantile conflicts aids and interprets the regression. In this sense, the utilization of a reductive approach is a purposive step in the individuation process.

> Regarded causally, regression is determined, say, by a "mother fixation." But from the final standpoint the libido regresses to the *imago* of the mother in order to find there the memory associations by means of which further development can take place, for instance from a sexual system into an intellectual or spiritual system.[43]

An individual working through infantile relationships with parental images is also working on personal individuation and the integration of archetypal issues. For example, the son afraid of abandonment by his mother clings to her instead of trying to develop. An analytic goal would be to help the patient become conscious of his infantile fears of loss and to develop a stable ego structure capable of functioning independently, so that separation from the mother can take place. All the countless affects, fears, projections and defenses inherent in this process will manifest in the transference. The analyst, as a result of projection, becomes the mother who does not want the son to separate and threatens abandonment. The analyst may even become the son afraid to separate while the patient becomes the abandoning mother who threatens to leave the analysis.

But this personal drama is not only a repetition of an early object-relationship, it is also a manifestation of the archetypal motif of the hero's struggle with the devouring aspect of the Great Mother. Just as the archetypal hero develops through stages such as son-lover, phallic hero, sun hero and so on, so the patient relives aspects of that archetypal drama in his personal transference dynamics. Similarly, other archetypal motifs and stages of development are experienced

---

[43] "On Psychic Energy," *The Structure and Dynamics of the Psyche,* CW 8, par. 43.

via the personal dynamics that manifest in the transference. Even when clinical considerations mitigate against mentioning archetypal issues and the transference is interpreted reductively and personalistically, the individuation process is taking place.

Whether an interpretation is causal or teleological, whether it deals with the progressive, developmental goals of the personality, depends not on whether it is reductive but on the perspective of the analyst. If the analyst experiences the momentary interpretation from the perspective of the analysand's potential development, then the particular intervention, whether synthetic or reductive, serves the analysand's individuation and is teleologically oriented.

Jung's writings on the subject of transference clearly indicate that, at least in its initial phases, transference should be analyzed reductively. The synthetic mode of interpretation does not begin until the causal-reductive mode ceases to bring new material to light and it becomes necessary to deal with archetypal motifs. But such cases are unusual.

With most patients, according to Jung, the application of the reductive approach will lead to the withdrawal of the personal infantile projections, and with the dissolution of the transference the analysis will terminate. The energy freed from the resolved transference neurosis moves into increased adaptation which, in most cases, satisfies the purpose of the neurosis. But if an exclusively personal, reductive approach is used then analysands might be left with the depressing experience that analysis has shown them to be nothing but a mass of relatively unresolved infantile conflicts. While this may be preferable to their previous condition, it would have failed to impart a sense that there was meaning and purpose to their illness and that it had been a necessary part of a developmental process.

The solution to this problem does not lie in the premature use of the synthetic method. Rather, I believe, the purposive orientation of the personality can be imparted by embedding reductive-causal interpretations in a final matrix that indicates the purposive function of the behavior being analyzed. The regressive infantile event can be treated both as symptom and as symbol.

For example, a male patient experienced difficulties in his relationships with women. His transference associations and fantasies clustered around the idea of oedipal competition. He wondered which of us had a larger penis, whether he or I earned more money, who had more girlfriends. The patient experienced frightening fantasies of my raping him in a homosexual rage. He also fantasized castrating me, chopping up my penis and using it as an ingredient in a stew.

As a reduction to a *causa efficiens,* these associations indicate that the patient's difficulties with women were related to a conflict with his father. This centered on competitive feelings, a desire to replace his mother and submit homosexually to his father, together with castration anxiety defended against by a fantasied castration of the father/analyst.

A reductive interpretation embedded in a purposive orientation would maintain that the patient's relational difficulties were connected to specific oedipal conflicts such as homosexual submission experienced as fear of rape, castration anxiety and so on. In addition, incorporative fantasies would be interpreted so as to indicate that his unconscious is presenting this material in the transference because the conflicts need to be resolved, so that the phallic potency necessary for the patient's individuation process can be liberated from its pathological fixation.

Which interpretive approach is used depends on clinical circumstances. With some patients, for instance those who experience pathological fears of success, any indication of a purposive attitude will arouse the patient's defenses. For these persons a strict reductive-causal method that analyzes the relationship between their infantile fears and their avoidance of success is necessary, at least initially. With others, for example those who suffer severe narcissistic pathology, reductive interpretation is experienced as a humiliating criticism from the idealized analyst. For such individuals, reductive interpretations are more easily accepted and integrated when embedded in a purposive matrix. In yet other situations, the archetypal, synthetic approach, or transference interventions that focus on the "here and now," are called for.

The value of the transference

One can only speculate on the reasons for Jung's contradictory standpoints about the significance of the transference. Some of

Jung's statements seem to be indicative of his personal conflicts with Freud. Transference was the centerpiece of Freud's therapeutic system and one of his most profound discoveries. By devaluing its significance, Jung may have been devaluing Freud, just as Freud denigrated Jung and his insights.

Perhaps this partially accounts for Jung's comment that he preferred no transference because he could then get all the necessary material from the dreams. Jung might have said this during "The Tavistock Lectures" because his audience wanted a talk on the transference rather than a continuation of his discourse on the amplification of dreams. However, one cannot use the same argument to account for Jung's similar remark in "The Psychology of the Transference." Here one does get the feeling that he preferred to work with dreams rather than with the transference.

In addition, one may speculate that Jung had difficulty in handling some aspects of the personal transference, which he experienced as obstacles to his work. Certainly there is enough recently published material to indicate that he experienced significant countertransference reactions, especially to the erotic component of the positive transference, which he found difficult to manage.[44] This may have led him to downplay the significance of the personal component of the transference and try to find other means of treating his patients.

According to much of Jung's writings on the subject, the transference functions psychologically in a manner similar to dreams. Both present material determined by the need to compensate the one-sided attitude of consciousness; both present unconscious material via projections, which contain a subjective and objective value; and both are purposive and serve the individuation process. Why, then, declare one a resistance and an obstacle and the other the preferred mode of treatment?

Finally, there are Jung's comments in "The Psychology of the Transference" about his preference for a mild rather than a strong

---

[44] See A. Carotenuto, *A Secret Symmetry: Sabina Spielrein Between Jung and Freud;* P. Stern, *C.G. Jung: The Haunted Prophet,* pp. 134-141; A. Storr, "Review of *A Secret Symmetry: Sabina Spielrein Between Jung and Freud*"; V. Brome, *Jung: Man and Myth,* p. 257; G. Wehr, *Jung: A Biography,* pp. 138-143, 187-190.

transference. Psychoanalysis in Jung's time was mainly a treatment for neurotic disorder. Diagnostically, strong transferences, especially early in an analysis, are often a sign of the severity of the patient's condition. It is only recently that there has developed an understanding of, and analytic procedures for treating, pre-oedipal conditions such as borderline disorders where intense, and often chaotic, transference reactions appear soon after treatment begins.[45] Jung's comments about preferring a mild to a severe transference may be based not only on his wish to have an easier time of it personally, but also on his clinical experience of the difficulty of treating those who early in analysis develop strong transferences.

With regard to the value of the transference, I prefer to give more weight to Jung's comments on its importance. They seem more reasoned and less contaminated by the emotional extremism of his contradictory statements which devalue the central position of the transference in analytic work. In addition, my experience is that analysis of the transference is the therapeutic lever that makes meaningful change possible. In that sense, it is indispensable for individuation.

---

[45] See J. Masterson, *The Narcissistic and Borderline Disorders;* O. Kernberg, *Borderline Conditions and Pathological Narcissism;* H. Spotnitz, *Psychotherapy of Preoedipal Conditions.*

2
The Therapeutic Utilization of Countertransference

The topic of countertransference is actually a subtopic of the idea of the wounded healer, an ancient and widespread image.[1] Chiron, the Centaur who taught Asclepius the healing arts, himself suffered from incurable wounds. In Babylon there was a dog-goddess with two names: as Gula she was death and as Labartu, healing. In India Kali is the goddess of the pox and at the same time its curer. Psychologically this means not only that the patient has a healer within, but also that the healer is wounded.

The psychotherapist is wounded in a number of ways. To begin with, those who enter the profession usually do so from an original position as suffering patient. Psychological pain causes future therapists to have to work extensively on their own wounds in order to live a satisfactory personal life. Some, often those who have had to spend the most time healing themselves, are called to psychological healing as a profession. Wounds, however, are seldom healed permanently. A vulnerability continues to exist which can be activated by close proximity to the wounds of others. In analytic work, the analyst's unconscious is penetrated by the patient's pain and the therapist becomes psychically infected by the projections to which he or she is exposed. Thus the healer is wounded again by taking on the illness of the other. This is especially the case when the patient's unconscious conflicts are in areas similar to those in which the therapist is scarred.

Being wounded is not just an inevitable and painful fate, it is also a necessary aspect of helping others. It is only through the knowledge derived from attempting to heal one's own wounds that the therapist can help others. In addition, the therapist does not not heal the other directly, but by arousing the healing process in the patient's

---

[1] See C.A. Meier, *Ancient Incubation and Modern Psychotherapy,* and C. Jess Groesbeck, "The Archetypal Image of the Wounded Healer."

unconscious. The analyst serves as a model of a healed person. This constellates the wounded healer archetype in the patient's unconscious, and that actually does the healing, not the analyst.

While there is renewed interest in the idea of the wounded healer, little has been said about the specific wounds the healer has to contend with and how they affect treatment. The psychological processes the analyst goes through in trying to derive meaning from inner experiences need to be more fully elaborated. In discussing these topics, my goal is to stimulate further discussion on how we, as analysts, utilize our reactions for the therapeutic benefit of our patients. To this end, I will present some ideas and insights relating to countertransference and illustrate them with examples from my own work with patients, from the work of those I have supervised, and from colleagues' experiences.

An important issue that will not be addressed here is the use the analyst makes of countertransference reactions in understanding his or her own personality. It is assumed that analysts are fragile human beings who recognize that lacunae exist and continue to struggle for self-understanding, often in their own on-going analysis. Given this, the question is, "Why do these particular countertransference reactions occur now and in relation to this particular person?"

The Useful Countertransference

Freud's original opinion of countertransference was similar to his view of transference; he considered it a hindrance to therapeutic progress. Unlike transference, which he ultimately came to see as not only inevitable but also necessary and valuable, Freud never altered his opinion about countertransference. To the end, he considered countertransference to be a sign of neurosis in the analyst that was to be avoided. It was not thought to provide useful information about the patient.

A major development in the concept of countertransference occurred when it began to be seen as a phenomenon of importance in helping the analyst to understand the hidden meaning of material brought by the patient. In psychoanalytic literature, the first explicit statement of the positive value of countertransference was made by

Paula Heimann in 1950.[2] She regarded countertransference as covering all the feelings experienced by analysts toward their patients. She maintained that analysts must use their emotional responses to patients as a key to understanding the patient. Her basic assumption was that the analyst's unconscious understands that of the patient. This rapport comes to the surface in the form of a feeling-response to the patient. Analysts have to be able to sustain the stirred up feelings, as opposed to discharging them, in order to subordinate them to the analytic task.

Jung, some fifteen years prior to Heimann, raised many of the same ideas. In "The Tavistock Lectures," Jung said that "any process of an emotional kind immediately arouses similar processes in others."[3] In therapy, the analyst will be affected by the patient's emotions and "he cannot do more than become conscious of the fact that he is affected. . . . It is even his duty to accept the emotions of the patient and to mirror them."[4]

In "The Psychology of the Transference," Jung developed this point further when he said that the analyst quite literally takes over and shares the sufferings of his patients.[5] The analyst's personal feelings, Jung argued, are then governed by those same unconscious contents that have become activated in the patient. This process provides a therapeutic opportunity if the analyst is able to make the transferred contents conscious. By understanding the activated material in oneself, it can be returned to the patient in a form that can be integrated.

From Jung's idea of the therapeutic value in the analyst's introjection of the patient's pathology, Fordham developed the concept of the "syntonic" countertransference. Fordham's concept is similar to Racker's idea of the "useful" countertransference and Adler's of the "true" countertransference.[6]

---

[2] "On Countertransference," pp. 81-84.

[3] *The Symbolic Life,* CW 18, par. 318.

[4] Ibid., par. 319.

[5] *The Practice of Psychotherapy,* CW 16, pars. 364-365.

[6] See M. Fordham, "Analytical Psychology and Countertransference," in *Countertransference;* H. Racker, *Transference and Countertransference;* G. Adler, *The Living Symbol.*

The premise behind these ideas is that, as a result of an unconscious effect, analysts become aware of reactions within themselves for which they cannot completely account in terms of their own psychology. These reactions become meaningful only when considered in terms of the patient's psychology. Constructive therapeutic intervention is an expression of an interchange in which psychic contents pass unconsciously from the patient to the analyst and then consciously from the analyst to the patient.

For example, during my first session with one woman, while she was talking about her abusive boyfriend, I suddenly had the frightening fantasy that he was outside the door and would come in and shoot us both. Later in the session the patient, with great shame, told me a dream in which she murdered her mother. I then realized that I had somehow become identified with her mother and feared the patient's murderous feelings which, in my fantasy, were projected onto the image of the boyfriend. Awareness of my countertransference fantasy helped me to understand the relationship between the patient's split-off rage and the abusive men she had become involved with. Months later, I could help her understand how she found and provoked abuse in men as a way of ridding herself of her own unacceptable rage and hate. The men became the carriers of this, while she, to avoid guilt, unconsciously identified with her mother who she imagined to be terrified of her daughter's murderous impulses.

Sometimes, as in this case, the analyst's countertransference reactions are clothed in images from the patient's material. Such reactions are readily experienced as having to do with the patient's psychology. At other times, however, the analyst's reactions may be clothed in personal images. These countertransference reactions often lead to resistance by the analyst because they are mistaken for personal reactions, and their significance for the patient may easily be overlooked. Close attention to the images or language of the fantasy often reveal distinguishing features not characteristic of the analyst's normal functioning. To understand such countertransference reactions the analyst needs to separate the themes of the countertransference fantasy from the concrete images in which they appear, just as the concrete images that archetypes clothe themselves in need to be separated from the archetypal themes they express.

For example, the woman mentioned above was silent for most of a session. Reflecting on her resistance, I recalled an earlier interpretation about her submissive behavior to her boss to which she had responded with defensiveness. I suggested she was angry at my previous observation and that her silence was an expression of this anger.

During the continued silence that followed this intervention, I fantasized being sexually dominant with a woman I knew. As I reflected on this fantasy a number of factors stood out: first, I do not enjoy sado-masochistic sexual domination; second, the woman in the fantasy was a friend who had recently, with great embarrassment, told me she was exploring the masochistic side of her personality and had discovered that it aroused her to be degraded; third, I did not feel aroused by the fantasy or experience any desire to act it out with my patient.

In my mind, the underlying theme that emerged, aside from the personal images that surfaced in me, was of someone who was ashamed of her desire to be sexually dominated. This, I concluded, was the basis for my patient's silent resistance. Rather than being angry at me, she was sexually aroused by some humiliation she had experienced—real or fantasized—at my hands, and was too self-conscious to reveal her reaction.

As I was thinking this, the patient suddenly blurted out that she knew I felt critical and angry toward her for the way she had been submitting to her boss. On the basis of my countertransference fantasy, I commented that her resistance may have been caused by her reaction to thoughts of me. With great distress she revealed that the thought of my yelling at her, dominating her like her boss, was sexually arousing. This reaction was analogous to her submission to her boss. Rather than being angry at her boss's domination, she realized she unconsciously provoked it in order to gain sexual satisfaction.

Some of the important psychological processes that the analyst uses in attempting to derive meaning from such countertransference experiences are empathy, trial identification and imagination. The analyst, through knowledge of the patient's psyche and his or her own imagination, empathically experiences the patient's world and allows his or her own psyche to react as the patient's psyche would. If the analyst has fewer defenses than the patient, the analyst's imagination will supply associations—images, feelings and thoughts—which indicate what is unconscious in the patient. This is a conscious process through which the analyst relates to his or her own unconscious in order to understand something about the other.

To illustrate, a trainee discussed a case concerning a woman, with whom he had a very good working relationship, who became hostile and withdrawn. She not only experienced herself as regressing, but questioned whether she had actually made any real progress in the analysis. At first, the trainee thought the patient's negative feelings were a reaction to his upcoming vacation. However, interpretations proved ineffective in bringing insight or altering her mood. After a number of weeks of fruitless work, the trainee noticed that he looked forward to her sessions with trepidation, even wishing she would cancel her hours due to illness. I suggested that he utilize these reactions as the basis for imaginal self-exploration. His fantasies indicated that he was afraid his patient would decide he was an unhelpful incompetent and abandon him. She would accuse him of not being able to help her understand what had precipitated her negative feelings or derive meaning from them. He felt inadequate, rejected and unloved by someone he needed value from. He also felt childish, imagining himself as about five years old.

For my part, I wondered whether the trainee's fantasy was a reflection of his patient's inner world; she might be feeling that he was dissatisfied with her progress in analysis, that he considered her inadequate as a patient and was preparing to reject her. The therapist then recalled an erotic countertransference reaction he had noticed and disregarded in response to a dream the patient had briefly mentioned a number of weeks prior. In the dream a teacher failed her because she could not speak fluent French. She had complained to the teacher that it was only the first class and that she could master the subject by the end of the course. The teacher left refusing to change her grade.

In her associations to the dream, the patient said that French was the language of romance. The trainee then intuitively understood that the patient was beginning to experience romantic and erotic feelings toward him and felt that he would be impatient with her development. In the transference, he had become her father who had withdrawn from her attempts at affection. In her young imagination she had blamed herself for his failure of feeling, accusing herself of being inadequate in comparison to her mother. The trainee's upcoming vacation was experienced as an abandonment caused by her budding romantic feelings. In her imagination he was going off with another woman, her mother, whom he experienced as more romantically adequate. With these insights the therapist was able to listen to her current associations with a new perspective and appropriately interpret the basis of her hurt and her retaliatory aggression.

These examples illustrate that, as a result of an unconscious effect, an analyst may perceive a patient's fantasies before the patient is conscious of them. Such countertransference experiences provide instructive information about the patient and the analytic relationship. However, it is often not therapeutic for the analyst to interpret information derived from the countertransference before the patient provides relevant material, indicating the fantasies are close to the surface and capable of being experienced. If the analyst interprets the countertransferentially understood material without relevant associations from the patient, the analyst is basically relying on intuition and authority to overcome the patient's defenses, rather than interpreting the patient's resistances.

My experience is that interventions are more useful when presented on the basis of the patient's material, not on the therapist's intuition. This does not mean that therapists do not use their intuition to understand the meaning their countertransference has for the patient, any more than they cease to utilize their other functions. Rather, therapists use their intuitive understanding of the countertransference to internally formulate what they think is unconsciously going on in the patient. But it is more therapeutic to contain such formulations until there is corroboration and an interpretative basis from the patient's material—such as dreams and associations.

Interpretations of the patient's unconscious processes that result solely from the analyst's intuitive understanding of countertransference are easily ignored, even if the patient consciously accepts them. If accepted, such interpretations unnecessarily increase irrational transference idealization by creating a magical aura about the analyst who can read the patient's mind. Furthermore, intuition can serve as a vehicle for the analyst's pathological projections onto the patient. Somehow, the analyst "knows" that the thoughts, feelings and impulses experienced in his or her own psychology are unconsciously perceived projections from the patient. This is a defensive use of intuition, an example of neurotic countertransference.

Neurotic Countertransference

What can be voluntarily experienced by the analyst about the patient is limited by the analyst's personal psychological development. If a particular subject arouses excessive anxiety and rejection in the analyst, he or she will not be able to empathically experience and identify that issue in the patient's unconscious. Instead, the analyst's neurotic conflicts distort both the perception and intervention. In such cases, the patient represents for the analyst an object of the past onto whom past feelings and wishes are projected, just as it happens in the patient's transference situation with the analyst.

Jung was one of the first analysts to recognize the difficulties that arise from the analyst's unresolved infantile conflicts. As early as 1912, he wrote that a successful analysis depended "on how far the analyst has been analyzed himself. If he himself has an infantile type of desire of which he is still unconscious, he will never be able to open his patient's eyes to this danger."[7]

In 1935, Jung observed that patients unconsciously attach their projections to similar vulnerabilities they sense in the analyst. He warned that the emotions of patients are "very contagious when the contents which the patient projects into the analyst are identical with the analyst's own unconscious contents."[8] At such times a state of *participation mystique* exists, a condition of mutual unconsciousness based on mutual projection, and allows no possibility of insight. Transference exists, but cannot be interpreted because the analyst is unconsciously colluding with the patient.

For example, a colleague hugged a particular patient at the end of every session. This practice had begun when, at the end of a stress-

---

[7] "The Theory of Psychoanalysis," *Freud and Psychoanalysis,* CW 4, par. 447.

[8] "The Tavistock Lectures," *The Symbolic Life,* CW 18, par. 322.

ful session involving the patient's recognition of the rage involved in her life-long depression, the patient asked for a hug. After the next session the patient again asked for a hug and, because of a counter-transference fear of the negative transference, the analyst again consented. The practice of the hug was born.

I suggested to my colleague that while his fear of the negative transference undoubtedly reflected some yet unresolved issue in his own psychology, there was also meaning in it for his patient. Since the hugging had begun after the patient began to become aware of her rage, it probably was a repetition of some earlier situation having to do with anger.

After the next session the patient again asked for a hug and the analyst suggested that rather than granting the request it should be discussed the following session. The next time she came the patient recalled that whenever she was angry as a child her mother eased her anger with a hug. She wanted the analyst to do the same. When he suggested that it would be more productive to allow the anger to emerge, the patient became enraged.

Over the next year she manifested an intense negative transference characterized by fantasies of the analyst being cold, afraid to show his feelings, disinterested and uncaring. As the patient recognized that her anger was accepted and had not destroyed the analyst, she recalled a repressed childhood perception that her mother was too fragile to handle the patient's aggression. She began to realize that her mother's hugs made her feel guilty and indicated her mother's unwillingness to allow the anger. The analyst's fear of not hugging the patient was an identification with the projection of the patient's mother. So long as it was acted out it could not be interpreted as a transference. Rather, the analyst was repetitively confirming to the patient that the patient's aggression was too terrifying to be consciously related to.

Fordham has further developed Jung's observations on the effects of the analyst's neurosis through his concept of countertransference "illusions," paralleled by Racker's concept of the "neurotic" counter-transference and Adler's idea of "counter-projection."[9] According to

---

[9] See above, note 6.

Fordham, countertransference illusions occur when analysts project their unconscious conflicts and then experience them as belonging to the patient. Conversely, the analysts may introject and identify with a part of the patient's unconscious.

The concept of projective identification is sometimes used in a defensive way by analysts to rationalize neurotic introjective identification. It is a variant of "he made me do it," and denies the fact that any prolonged introjective identification—indeed, any identification that is compulsively acted out—is a result of the patient's projection arousing a corresponding problem in the analyst.

Fordham considers projections and introjections that result in identifications as the worst obstruction to analysis. They result in a denial of the patient's true identity and manipulative attempts by the analyst to make the patient fit the analyst's illusion.

While it is generally agreed that neurotic countertransference is harmful, the idea has developed that it may nevertheless provide helpful information about the patient. Naturally, there is a reluctance by analysts to admit to and explore the painful and embarrassing fact of their own neurosis and its effects on the patient. That such opprobrium still exists is evidenced by the paucity of literature on this subject. Recently, however, there seems to be a greater willingness among analytic authors to acknowledge their neurotic reactions to analysands. Langs and Searles have both examined the effect of neurotic countertransference on the patient and the patient's attempts to communicate perceptions of the analyst's neurosis:

> Consciously, and more usually unconsciously, the patient perceives and detects the analyst's problems, takes them into himself through introjective identification or refuses to contain them, and at times, becomes involved in efforts to cure the analyst through a modification of the pathological introjects and through direct, usually unconscious confrontations and interpretations. Silently—and humbly— the analyst can greatly benefit from these efforts, without specifically acknowledging their presence.[10]

A discrimination of the broad category of neurotic countertransfer-

---

[10] R. Langs, *The Therapeutic Interaction: A Synthesis,* p. 122; H.F. Searles, "The Patient As Therapist to His Analyst."

ence into subgroups has developed. Langs has differentiated neurotic countertransference into acute and characterological forms.[11] Reich says that acute countertransferences

> are those which occur suddenly, under specific circumstances and with specific patients. . . . One is faced with counter-transference reactions which are provoked by the specific content of the patient's material. . . . Sometimes the disturbances are of a more general nature, not dependent on any special situation of the analyst or special material. . . . Such manifestations of counter-transference . . . reflect permanent neurotic difficulties of the analyst.[12]

Stein follows their general classification and adds an additional helpful category of countertransference phases: longer periods of countertransference patterns that an analysis goes through.[13]

Characterological countertransferences are an expression of the analyst's general character problems that permeate the entire work. For example, an analyst with unconscious aggression may continuously project aggressive motives onto patients, or the analyst's interpretations may be made in a hostile and critical manner. On the other hand, the analyst may overcompensate and become excessively supportive. Other characterological problems include unconscious narcissistic conflicts that may cause an analyst to look to the patient for admiration or to overevaluate therapeutic progress. Characterological countertransferences are recalcitrant to modification through self-analysis and, when pointed out by an analysand or colleagues, result in denial and defense by the analyst.

Acute countertransference reactions are easier to address. While they are often acted out, the analyst soon realizes something has gone wrong and does not need to defend against understanding. Frequently, self-analysis or discussion with a supervisor or colleague can resolve the problem. After the analyst has gained control of the reaction's neurotic aspect, acknowledged the pathology to oneself and, if it has been acted out, to the patient, the question arises of what it says about the particular patient.

---

[11] *The Therapeutic Interaction,* pp. 110-112.

[12] A. Reich, "On Countertransference," pp. 25-31.

[13] M. Stein, "Power, Shamanism and Maieutics in the Countertransference."

To effectively utilize the acute neurotic countertransference, the analyst's irrational responses must be understood as a combination of his or her own neurosis and that of the patient. Following Jung's suggestion that the analytic relationship be viewed as a commingling of both psyches, the analyst's countertransference can be considered a combination of the analyst's own tendencies and a reflexive acceptance of the role projected by the patient.

In the transference, patients tend to repeat rather than remember past pathogenic experiences and thereby engage the analyst in a re-enactment of the past. The patient tries to manipulate the analyst into playing a role complementary to the one the patient experiences and then unconsciously adapts to the perceived reaction. If the analyst is not aware of it, he or she will tend to comply. Rather than an analysis of the patient's transferred past, the process is a repetition, with the same destructive effects. While the analyst must always take responsibility for the neurotic element that caused the countertransference to be acted out, the behavior can still usefully be viewed as a combination of the analyst's own tendencies and the role relationship which the patient is unconsciously trying to establish.

In a session a number of years ago, my previously mentioned female patient was recounting a series of self-destructive incidents that had occurred during the week. This litany of woe culminated in a description of a self-destructive experience with a man, and she commented that she would continue to behave like this in order to hold on to him. During this tale my anger had been rising and after this last comment I began aggressively questioning her self-destructiveness. Afterward, I felt relieved, entirely justified, and convinced myself that I had done this questioning for her own good. I rationalized that my motivation had been to shake up her ego and to constellate the hero archetype to do battle with the regressive aspects of the unconscious.

A dream of mine a few days later led me to the painful conclusion that my motivations were not so pure. I realized that my behavior was a function of my own unintegrated power drive and a frustrated narcissistic image of myself as a magical healer. The analysand's resistance and associations next session allowed me an opportunity to interpret and confirm her feelings of having been bullied. The acknowledgment of my countertransference reaction diminished her resistance and allowed her to associate to the incident. She realized its similarity to other relationships in which she was abused and finally came to the insight that, when she felt threatened by feelings of abandonment, she unconsciously used her masochism to cling. She did this by constellating the other's abusive anger and then offering herself as an object of abuse. Thus, she hooked other people into continuing to relate to her via their need to have an object against which to express their rage. In our relationship she had been unconsciously afraid I would reject her because of her regressive behavior during the previous week. Unconsciously she led me into needing her as an object of abuse by arousing my hostility.

Obviously, it would have been more therapeutic for her if I had not acted out the abusive response. In any event, I was able to take responsibility for the unresolved conflicts that led me to act out this role; the interaction could then be explored for information about the patient that ultimately supported therapeutic progress.

The question arises, what factors might lead an analyst to conclude that a countertransference reaction is primarily a combination of the analyst's neurosis and that of the patient?

To personalize the issue: What assurance did I have that the first two fantasies I reported under the useful countertransference were not an indication of my own problem with the abusive use of power, while the most recently described situation was a combination of her self-destructive needs and an unresolved limitation of my own?

The first necessity is the analyst's awareness of his or her own psychology. Thanks to my personal analysis, I was confident in my ability ultimately to be aware of what belonged to me and what did not. This of course does not mean that I have no destructive potential. But the first two situations were not the type to stimulate that potential in a neurotic way. Rather it was through my aggressive potential that I could allow my countertransference fantasies to manifest and be observed. In contrast, incidents that affect my narcissism do have the potential to arouse hostility in me. This was the case in the latter example, where my frustration over not being able to help the patient combined with her need to arouse my aggression.

Second, as mentioned earlier, the quality of the fantasies in the first two instances—the one about the abusive boyfriend and the one about sexual dominance—were uncharacteristic for me but were characteristic of the patient.

Third, in the first two instances I felt no anxiety or defensiveness in allowing my fantasies to enter consciousness. I could calmly observe my inner life in reaction to the analysand. Most important, there was no impulse to act on the fantasies, either to behave in an abusive manner, to accuse her of trying to provoke me, or to bring the matter to a head in order to relieve myself of tension. By contrast, in the third example, I impulsively questioned her in an aggressive manner, felt self-righteous, defended myself to myself via rationalization, dreamed about the incident, and felt guilty about my reaction.

The Archetypal Countertransference

In chapter one, it was shown that the transference is archetypal in two ways: archetypal contents are projected onto the analyst, and the transference process itself is archetypal in that a purposive development toward individuation is inherent in it. Similarly, archetypal contents are aroused in the countertransference and there can be discerned a purpose and direction to the process.

During the process of individuation a person goes through a series of experiences of increasing unity between ego and unconscious, symbolized by images of the coniunctio. These experiences are mediated through the analytic relationship.

The first coniunctio is the encounter with the shadow. The contents of the shadow are projected not just because the psychic system defensively rids itself of painful inner stimuli, but because the drive for individuation demands that the unconscious be integrated, and projection is the means to that end. Since many of the personal contents of the shadow are made up of repressed or otherwise defended experiences which manifest in the transferences, the analysis of the transference is a significant step in the individuation process.

While personal conflicts about love and hate, desire and fear are analyzed reductively and causally so that the individual can become conscious of their determining influences, there is also a prospective or purposive value to this reduction. The negative transference, for instance, represents not only the projection of the patient's infantile conflicts over aggression, but also the need to separate from bondage to the parental imagos as the initial step in individual development.

For Jung, the negative transference is not only "an infantile wish for insubordination; it is a powerful urge to develop [one's] own personality, and the struggle for this is . . . an imperative duty."[14] By repeating in the analytic relationship the previously unsuccessful separation stages of early life, there occurs a renewed opportunity to differentiate from the unconscious identification with parental values and proceed into adulthood.

Similarly, Jung suggests that the positive transference is not just a projection of infantile-erotic fantasies, but serves the goal of uniting the patient with the analyst so that development of new, healthier adaptations can take place. Jung recognized the positive transference and countertransference as symbolic of the need for union between conscious and unconscious, with the analyst experiencing and representing the projected unconscious of the patient. It is only in the positive transference-countertransference that integration can occur. The erotic aspect of the transference-countertransference relationship is thus a symbol for the coniunctio and leads to wholeness.

On the level of the personal unconscious, the positive and negative transferences reflect particular conditioning of the instincts of love and aggression, but there is also an archetypal basis for these valences. With some analysands the archetypal transferences indicate fundamental conflicts over the existence of good and evil in the universe, underlying the personally toned conflicts. Correspondingly, the archetypal shadow countertransference indicates to the analyst that not only is a personal conflict present but that there is also a teleological meaning inherent in the conflict that points to the individuation needs of the analysand.

Edward Edinger suggests that evil constitutes a dark, unconscious side of the Self that needs to be made conscious by man's personal moral struggle.[15] In this sense, the individual's relationship to the dark side of the shadow, for instance primitive impulses of desire

---

[14] "Some Crucial Points in Psychoanalysis (Jung-Loÿ Correspondence)," *Freud and Psychoanalysis,* CW 4, par. 658.

[15] *The Creation of Consciousness: Jung's Myth for Modern Man,* chapt. 3.

and rage, is not only a personal issue, but an aspect of the archetypal drama of a coming to consciousness of the dark side of the Self.

An analyst with a comfortable relationship to the shadow will have a very different countertransference reaction than will one who is alienated from the shadow. The archetypal countertransference of the shadow is often threatening because the analyst begins to incarnate absolute evil unmitigated by human goodness, and this may arouse intense feelings of guilt and moral inferiority. Such reactions can be especially painful to those of a strict religious persuasion, due to the split between good and evil with which they have often identified.

One analyst, a former minister, had particular difficulty dealing with negative transferences from his patients. He would respond with defensive declarations that attempted to show he was not as they imagined. He became increasingly distressed with one analysand who developed the almost delusional idea that the analyst was an agent of the devil sent to corrupt him. The analyst could not talk his patient out of this idea.

I suggested that his inability to tolerate the patient's negative fantasies and use them as the basis for exploring the patient's shadow indicated some difficulty in accepting his own shadow. That night the analyst dreamed: "God, through the robe of the devil, visited me with a perversion to last through eternity." His dream helped him begin to come to terms with the idea that both good and evil existed in the universe and that evil was another manifestation of God. Only after this process had begun could he tolerate his patient's projection of evil onto him.

Any archetype that is aroused will affect the analyst's feelings about the patient. Archetypal countertransferences can be useful or destructive, depending on the analyst's relationship to the particular content constellated in his or her unconscious. The savior or the nurturing aspect of the Great Mother are common positive archetypal countertransference reactions. If the analyst is not conscious of the effects of these archetypes, the desire to help can induce the analyst to take exceptional responsibility for the care of the patient and cause guilt if the patient's condition does not improve. On the other hand, such countertransferences can lead to consciousness of archetypal dynamics activated in the patient. It is the analyst's awareness of the patterns of behavior and development inherent in archetypal energy that allows him or her to mediate the relationship between the patient's ego and the activated archetype.

Since it would be impossible to differentiate every possible archetypal image that can affect the analyst, I will instead indicate some criteria for differentiating archetypal from personal countertransferences. There is an experiential difference between the two which makes the archetypal countertransference especially difficult. Some personal countertransference reactions to transference idealization will illustrate this.

During the tenth analytic session with a new patient, I drew a parallel between a current relationship and one the analysand had had with his mother. He responded with silence, during which I had the following fantasy: Behind a one-way mirror in my office sat all the senior Jungian analysts in New York City. They were discussing the brilliance of my interpretation and the general excellence with which I was handling the case.

Reflecting on this fantasy, I realized that I really considered neither my interpretation nor my handling of the case brilliant. Quite the contrary, I was feeling confused and inept. I concluded that the fantasy must have been stimulated by an idealization occurring in the analysand. More to the immediate point, while my countertransference reaction was somewhat intense, the imagery was strictly personal, and while my pride was exaggerated it was not numinous; that is, I was great, but not godlike.

With the archetypal countertransference, the numinosity of the archetype often leads the analyst into an identification which is qualitatively and quantitatively different from the personal countertransference identifications. This is not exclusively due to unresolved narcissistic problems in the analyst. Adolf Guggenbühl-Craig suggests that because of the analyst's involvement with dreams and other manifestations of the unconscious, the archetypal image of the wise man and the priest are projected onto the analyst.[16] These constellated images are an occupational hazard, especially for Jungians. Archetypal imagery replaces personal imagery and the numinosity

---

[16] *Power in the Helping Professions,* pp. 20-35.

aroused resonates seductively in the analyst's psyche. The analyst who identifies too closely may actually think he or she is more deeply initiated into the secrets of the meaning of life and death than other mortals.

I remember a personal experience that illustrates this. On a hot summer day a number of years ago, I wore white clothes to my office. A patient told me I looked like a guru and in fact had long felt that I actually was a master. While I made an obligatory comment about it only being a projection, in fact I was secretly pleased and became identified with the image of the master. I pontificated quite proudly about many subjects related to the nature of existence, not only till the end of that session but for two sessions afterward. I finally disidentified from the priestly archetype over lunch when I took a bite out of my hamburger and ketchup squirted on my white shirt. This experience brought me back to my more mundane state and a realization of my all too human ridiculousness.

In dealing with the archetypal countertransference a sense of humor about oneself is mandatory. In addition, the objective level of interpretation should be utilized with great skepticism because of the danger that the analyst, the object of the patient's fantasies, will identify with, and attempt to retain, the patient's projections.

This danger is especially acute with archetypal variations of the positive transference. If the transference is of an erotic nature, the analyst may develop the fantasy that he or she can magically heal by sexual intercourse with the patient. In other instances, an analyst with unresolved narcissistic problems may insist on interpreting the patient's archetypal idealization on the objective level, with the analyst thereby becoming an object of worship. Similarly, an analyst with an unresolved savior complex will readily identify with the common projection of the savior archetype. One protection against identification with the archetypal content is the synthetic technique of amplifying the patient's images. Even silently citing the parallels can help the analyst recognize the transference image as a general and not personal phenomenon.

3

The Erotic and Aggressive Countertransferences

If it is accepted that through the understanding of countertransference analysts are provided with a therapeutic instrument of great value, the question turns to the meaning analysts can derive from these experiences. One of the current research tasks of Jungian psychology is to differentiate countertransference reactions so that individual analysts, working in isolation, may have a number of hypotheses to help them understand their reactions. For this process, unfortunately, there is little guidance in Jung's writings.

Contemporary analysts, however, have begun to explore this problem. Among Jungians, Adolf Guggenbühl-Craig describes how the archetypes of the healer, priest and savior affect transference-countertransference dynamics.[1] Marion Woodman differentiates the various stages of transference and countertransference that may develop with women who suffer from eating disorders.[2] Nathan Schwartz-Salant examines countertransference reactions to the personal and archetypal energies involved in the idealizing and mirror transferences characteristic of narcissistic disorders.[3] Murray Stein describes the dynamic interactions occurring around issues of power, shamanism and analytic midwifery.[4]

Such studies indicate that there are no obvious one-to-one relationships between the analyst's experience and the patient's inner life. Rather there exists a great complexity and difficulty in determining the meaning to be derived for the patient from the analyst's countertransference. Some of these issues will be explored here.

---

[1] *Power in the Helping Professions.*

[2] "Transference and Countertransference in Analysis Dealing with Eating Disorders."

[3] *Narcissism and Character Transformation: The Psychology of Narcissistic Character Disorders.*

[4] "Power, Shamanism, and Maieutics in the Countertransference."

The Erotic Countertransference

During a session an analyst may experience a sexual response toward a patient. Some of the possible meanings the analyst may derive from this are as follows.

1. Jung observed that an analyst's sexual response may indicate a compensation for poor rapport with the patient.[5] Personally, neither as a clinician nor as a clinical supervisor have I ever encountered an instance where the analyst's sexual response was solely compensatory to poor rapport. Rather, the analyst's sexual feelings are often a compensation for a poor relationship combined with other factors, such as unsatisfied sexual needs or the repression of sexuality in either analyst or patient.

For instance, an analyst-in-training dreamed that he and his female patient were lying on the floor of his office kissing passionately. He had developed an intense sexual countertransference and felt he loved her. He had fantasies of running off with her and imagined the two of them walking romantically on the beach. As he discussed the case it became clear that prior to his dream he had felt disconnected to his patient. He had blamed her resistance for his lack of interest, had lamented her inability to make progress and had considered terminating the analysis.

In this case the analyst's erotic countertransference overcompensated for his disinterest. It diminished when he began to understand and appreciate his patient. In addition to overcompensation, however, it also became clear that the analyst's loss of interest correlated to the patient's resistance to the development of an erotic transference. The analyst's dream, in turn, was stimulated by the patient's repressed sexuality which the analyst countertransferentially experienced and misidentified as his own. A further complicating factor indicated by the dream was the analyst's poor rapport with his own anima, compensated by his sexual countertransference, which was then defended against by a disinterest in the patient.

2. The analyst's sexual feelings toward the patient may indicate personal sexual deprivation. The analyst may not be neurotic about the subject of sexuality, but simply unconscious of the effects of his

---

5 "The Tavistock Lectures," *The Symbolic Life,* CW 18, par. 331.

or her unsatisfied needs. One male analyst interpreted all of a new female patient's material in terms of sexuality. In fact, she was very inhibited sexually and the analyst, through his aroused sexuality, was accurately picking up her conflicts. What he overlooked was that the patient was being traumatized by the discussion of sexuality so early in the analysis. After exploring his therapeutic approach in supervision and personal analysis, the analyst, whose wife had been working in a distant city for some time, understood that he was projecting his own unmet needs onto the patient.

3. The analyst's response may be related to his or her own neurosis. For example, one woman became sexually aroused whenever a male patient began to weep. This reaction was absent with female patients. Discussion revealed unconscious sadistic fantasies about men's pain and its ability to arouse her. A male analyst, with a similar reaction toward female patients, discovered it was related to narcissistic fantasies involving his hope to ease his patient's sufferings through the healing power of his phallus. In each of these instances, further personal analysis indicated the fantasies were related primarily to the analyst's unresolved conflicts.

Analysts who are afraid of their sexuality or think it neurotic and inappropriate to have a sexual response toward their patients, will communicate this unconsciously. For example, an older female analyst considered unethical her sexual attraction toward a young, attractive but inhibited male patient. Her anxiety caused her to change the subject and otherwise avoid his attempts to discuss his sexual conflicts. One night the patient dreamed that the analyst felt sexually aroused during a session and ran out of the room. Hesitantly, he associated to the dream feelings he had concerning the need to protect the analyst by not becoming sexually aroused himself. In her own analysis she realized that her sexual reaction to the patient created anxiety because of unconscious oedipal feelings toward her son projected onto the young man.

4. The analyst's sexual response may be aroused by a patient's conscious or unconscious seductiveness—dressing, acting or speaking in a provocative manner. The countertransference reaction can alert the analyst to this issue and lead to a better understanding of the patient's motivations. Perhaps the patient compensates for a feeling

of helplessness by sexual control; or the seduction may be a test of the analyst's ability to handle the patient's sexuality; or it may be a way the patient attempts to feel valued.

5. The analyst's sexual response may be an unconscious perception of the patient's repressed, undeveloped and, perhaps, initially stirring sexuality. In this sense the countertransference may be a purposive harbinger of the patient's future development. The analyst may not even mention the subject but, by consciously carrying the sexual experience, unconsciously communicate the acceptability of the patient's sexuality.

A number of years ago I worked with a woman who had spent her entire life in parochial schools. She was shy, inhibited and dominated by a strict father complex that criticized any display of instinctual life. Yet every time she entered my office I felt sexually stimulated and correspondingly guilty and could find no rational basis for either reaction. It was only after I heard a few of her dreams that I understood the unconscious connection.

In one dream, in the shadow of her inhibited conscious attitude lived a dark-haired French nightclub singer who wore a low cut black gown and was full of sexual vitality and seduction. Her boyfriend in the dream was a Robin Hood hero who lived by his wits outside traditional boundaries. Since this masculine figure corresponded to a then unconscious aspect of my own personality, I was all too ready to identify with her projection. While the conscious relationship was between myself as analyst and her as inhibited patient, the unconscious relationship was between her seductive sexual shadow and the dashing animus boyfriend that I had identified with. All of this, at first, went on quite unconsciously, except for the irrational sexual reaction and guilt I experienced. Understanding the countertransference not only revealed the shadow and animus relationship but also led to an understanding of the resistance. The guilt I felt over my sexual reaction was due to another identification, this time with her father complex, which condemned my sexual reaction the same as it condemned hers. Thus, both of us were involved in trying to repress our sexuality in order to placate her father complex rather than trying to make it conscious and analyze it.

6. The analyst's sexual response may be a concretization of a

symbolic event. In "The Transcendent Function," Jung wrote that the individual unconsciously attempts to bring about change through the union of conscious and unconscious.[6] Elsewhere Jung observed that relationship with an external other is a necessary ingredient for transformation because the unconscious needs an object on which to project its contents.[7] The analytic relationship mediates the transcendent function when unconscious contents projected onto the analyst are experientially understood and returned to the patient in a form that can be consciously integrated.

Jung also noted that the urge toward wholeness has an erotic aspect.[8] The symbol of the coniunctio, underlying both the archetypal drive toward union of conscious and unconscious as well as the transference-countertransference relationship, may be experienced concretely through the aroused sexuality of the participants; that is, there is a physical concomitant to the symbolic experience. This means that whenever the patient integrates an aspect of the unconscious which has been mediated via the transference-countertransference, there is the potential for eroticism. Through lack of understanding or neurosis, the analyst may misinterpret the symbolic expression of the patient's need for individuation and feel pressed to act out the erotic aspect of the coniunctio.[9] Where the pressure is not resisted, it would be a grave error to rationalize the acting out as a religious necessity performed at the behest of the Self or in the service of the patient's individuation.

The Aggressive Countertransference

Both positive and negative countertransferences present valuable information about the analysand's unconscious conflicts. Whether the presence of a countertransference indicates a healthy or pernicious development, and especially whether the analyst can derive meaning

---

[6] *The Structure and Dynamics of the Psyche,* CW 8, pars. 131-146.

[7] "The Psychology of the Unconscious," *The Practice of Psychotherapy,* CW 16, par. 454.

[8] Ibid., par. 460.

[9] For further discussion, see Mario Jacoby, *The Analytic Encounter: Transference and Human Relationship,* chapt. 5, "Erotic Love in Analysis."

from his or her inner reactions which can then be of therapeutic benefit to the patient, depends on the clinical circumstances. Some of the possible meanings the analyst may derive from an aggressive countertransference reaction are as follows.

1. The analyst's anger may indicate the patient's fear of intimacy and love.

Warm feelings toward the analyst may lead to the development of a positive working alliance which exposes the patient to deeper self-exploration and the discovery of pathological unconscious contents that have been avoided. The patient may also fear loving feelings because of concomitant sexual arousal. The erotic component of the positive transference causes particular difficulties when the analyst and analysand are of the same sex. Under such circumstances patients often dread any affectionate feelings toward the analyst because of fears of homosexuality.

Patients afraid of love try to find ways to maintain their aggressive feelings as a defense. Often they will attempt to manipulate the analyst into negative reactions or other inappropriate behavior so they can find valid reasons for distrust. For example, the patient may try to get the analyst to break the frame, reveal personal information or get angry.

Under such circumstances, the analyst's aggression toward the patient will derive from two sources. On the one hand, the analyst may introject the patient's defensive aggression and feel annoyed at the patient as well as affectionate. Self-analysis will often reveal the analyst's warm feelings, and the anger will be recognized as alien and belonging to the patient. The juxtaposition of anger and warmth in the analyst provides clues to the defensive process in the patient.

Shortly before I was to leave on a vacation I felt angry toward a patient. In reflecting on my feelings I was aware that while I was happy to be going away, I also liked working with this man, would genuinely miss him while I was gone and would be glad to see him when I returned. During the following session he presented a dream in which he was reunited with an old girlfriend. His associations to the dream included a movie in which a divorced couple remarried, and his mother's aborting a pregnancy in an earlier marriage. My interpretive response pointed to the patient's hopeful feelings of being reunited with me, as with an old girlfriend, and his fear that I, like his mother, would abandon (abort) him. His anger from the previous session was a defense against frightening feelings of love and possible abandonment. My negative feelings were an introjection of his defensive hostility.

On the other hand, a patient's need to justify defensive anger may result in behavior designed to provoke the analyst.

A training candidate came to a supervision session in great distress and described the following situation: An older patient said that he had never felt closer to anyone. This was very gratifying to the therapist who had put a great deal of effort into establishing a positive relationship. At the end of the session the patient informed him that he was cutting down his sessions from two to one a week. When the therapist asked the reason for such an abrupt change, the patient responded that their agreement called for the payment of missed sessions. The patient was going away on two business trips the following month and did not want to pay for sessions he would miss. He would cut down to once a week for one month and the following month would return to twice a week.

The analyst was shocked, especially in light of the tremendous effort he had made on the patient's behalf and the feelings of closeness expressed earlier by the patient. The analyst lost his temper and called the patient a psychopath. The patient responded that the analyst was solely interested in the money and he did not want to work with someone who would get so angry. During the week the patient left a message on the analyst's answering machine terminating the analysis.

2. The analyst's anger may be indicative of the patient's angry feelings, which the patient either does not consciously recognize or is too frightened to express directly.

One of the characteristics of neurosis is a diminished capacity to contain the ambivalence due to internal conflict; one side remains unconscious and does not mitigate the other. As a result of this breakdown in compensation there develops an extreme and unrealistic attitude. An analytic goal under such circumstances is to present the unconscious position to the patient in order to initiate a compensating alternation which may result in a more realistic perspective.

A persistent and extreme positive attitude toward the analyst is often an indication of unconscious hostility. Jung recognized that when the rapport between analyst and patient is unsatisfactory, the unconscious of either patient or analyst may compensate with an intensified erotic transference.[10] The reverse is also true. When the relationship between the analyst and patient is too good, when there is too much positive feeling, the analyst's unconscious may respond with anger as a way of bringing the unrecognized negative aspect of the relationship into consciousness.

I once worked with a man who always came on time, paid his bills promptly, expressed great appreciation for my help and generally enhanced my security. After a personal dream in which I felt angry toward this patient, I realized that the relationship was too good. During sessions subsequent to my dream, I found ways to indicate to the patient that the relationship was one-sided in its feeling tone. The patient realized he worked well in order to gain my love and that his cooperativeness was a form of submission similar to the manifest compliance he had with his father. His positive feelings were a defense against the negative transference. After the defensive aspect of his positive working alliance was worked through, the patient became enraged not only at himself for being so submissive, but also at me for fostering this submissive alliance in order to help him get better. Now he was determined to have a bad relationship, not accept any of my interpretations and not get better.

It is often difficult to uncover the patient's aggressive feelings, not only because the patient resists the recognition of his or her hate, fear and suspicion, but also because the analyst may collude, consciously or unconsciously, with the patient's utilization of loving feelings for defensive purposes. This is especially the case when the patient's anger is due not to transference fantasies, but to valid perceptions of inappropriate behavior by the analyst. The patient may recognize the analyst's error but be afraid to mention it. Or transference factors may inhibit the patient's conscious realization, but dreams and associations indicate an unconscious awareness of an error or some weakness in the analyst.

---

10 "The Therapeutic Value of Abreaction," *The Practice of Psychotherapy*, CW 16, par. 276.

A colleague had a policy of charging analysands for missed appointments. A relatively new patient with whom he had made this agreement went on a business trip and, out of a countertransference fear of eliciting a negative transference, the analyst promised to make up the two sessions the patient would miss. After his return, the analyst made up one session and then, conveniently, did not have time to make up the other. The patient never mentioned it but they continued to have what seemed like a good rapport. However, my colleague noticed a prolonged emptiness and superficiality to the patient's associations and a lack of significant progress in their work. The analyst's frustration and annoyance led me to suggest that he reassess the patient's dreams and associations in terms of anger. I pointed out the patient's many references to figures in his life who were unreliable, dishonest and sloppy in their work habits. I suggested that the patient had displaced his hostile feelings onto external figures and he and the analyst were colluding in being angry at them, rather than realizing the patient's anger toward the analyst.

In this case, the analyst had to be careful not to interpret the patient's anger as a displaced transference; rather, the patient's reaction was based on his objective observation that the analyst had proven himself unreliable. What could be interpreted as due to a transference fantasy was the way the patient handled his appropriate hostile reaction. Rather than recognizing and confronting the analyst with his feelings, the patient's fear of rejection caused him to defensively displace his angry reaction onto other figures. Only after persistent interpretation of his negative feelings and rectification by the analyst, that is, making up the missed session, was the analysis able to progress.

3. The analyst's anger may be an expression of his own acute or chronic neurotic countertransference.

Unresolved guilt over anger may lead an analyst to resist recognizing it. Such feelings can often be identified by their derivatives, which manifest alongside the positive countertransference. Stopping the session early or starting it late, wishing the patient would miss appointments, not billing on time, frequent glances at the clock, yawning or using confrontation as a dominant interpretive technique may all indicate repressed anger. Submissive, masochistic behavior on the part of the analyst often indicates an underlying fear of the analyst's own hostility. Similarly, anxiety reactions often derive from projected hostility.

During supervision, one analyst interspersed subtle hostile comments within her case presentation and denied their significance when they were brought to her attention. After the analyst commented "jokingly" that the patient's attempt to study Chinese was due to the desire to open a Chinese laundry, I suggested that her comment was an indication of her anger toward the patient. She protested and continued the "joke" by saying she really meant that the patient planned to open a Chinese restaurant.

In her personal analysis, this therapist subsequently discovered that she experienced the patient's study of Chinese as a narcissistic attack. She was particularly vulnerable to feelings of inadequacy which she defended against through control. Seeing her patient improve made her feel competent. Since the patient considered Chinese to be the most difficult language and the Chinese people to be superior, the analyst considered the patient's study of Chinese a regressive act of defensive superiority. The analyst felt angry at the patient for getting worse, especially after the patient's previous improvement had helped the analyst feel successful. Now the analyst felt let down, helpless, responsible, and blamed the patient in order to preserve her own feelings of self-worth.

4. The analyst's anger may be due to the introjection of various structures in the patient's personality.

As a result of the unconscious connection between analyst and patient the analyst may internally experience the patient's conflicted inner relationships.

On the one hand, the analyst may feel the desire to behave toward the patient as significant others from the patient's past have. For example, the patient may project a dominating father onto the analyst and respond with fear, submission or rebelliousness. People who project an oedipal father often act in a frustrating or competitive way. If the analyst identifies with the projected oedipal father, he or she may try to overpower and dominate the patient with interpretations.

Conversely, the analyst may feel treated by the patient as the patient was in the past, especially if the patient currently identifies with a significant other. In these circumstances, the feelings, attitudes and values associated with the patient's childhood ego are transferred to the analyst. For example, the patient may have a desire to express angry feelings toward perceived slights from the analyst. Because of fear of the transferred punitive parents the ego desire to be angry may be repressed and projected onto the analyst. The patient may then identify with the values of the punitive parents and attack the analyst for advocating hostile behavior.

5. The analyst's anger may be a harbinger of future developments in the patient.

Anger in a patient is often a preliminary reaction to necessary separations and growing self-assertion. The analyst's anger can be a reflection of this. For instance, a dependent patient whose dreams indicated an unconscious rebelliousness toward his mother started the session with the following comments.

"I'm thinking of ending the analysis this August. I've gained a lot from it, but it's five years now and at some point I have to go out on my own. I know you'll think it's a resistance but I don't. . . . My mother called the other day and hassled me about the new vacation house I'm buying. She's still trying to control me even though I'm a grown man. I should have told her to mind her own business. . . . My wife and I had a fight last weekend over who would get their way in regard to different movies we each wanted to see. I feel like finding another woman and having an affair. . . . I was watching a television show in which a woman who had been submissive all her life finally asserted her independence and left her husband. Now she'd have freedom to live her own life. But he wasn't really trying to dominate her and would have let her change if she stayed."

These comments helped me realize that an unaccountable anger I had been experiencing toward this man was related to an aggressive force preparing to manifest in his own psyche. It helped me prepare for the transferential expression of his self-assertion through conflicts such as threats of separation and the rejection of all my interventions, and helped me maintain the perspective that his aggression was developmental and in the service of his individuation process.

4
The Fear of Therapeutic Progress

Jungian psychology has tended to overemphasize the integrative, progressive aspect of the unconscious. Analysts like to view the unconscious as the creative matrix of life which, if properly understood and integrated, can direct one toward future growth. After all, inherent in the symbols we so love to interpret is a developmental directive: the path toward individuation, the path to wholeness.

Implicit is the assumption that so long as the direction of psychological growth is clearly evident in the symbols produced by the unconscious, the inherent need for individuation will cause the individual to choose that way. Presumably, the analyst's job is to help make evident the patient's developmental path by interpreting symbols, supporting the creative forces of the unconscious and encouraging the integration of the disparate parts of the patient's personality.

What may be forgotten is that alongside, and in opposition to, the forces stimulating psychological growth, there exists a fear of it. Jung attributed this fear to an instinctive regressive force inherent in the psyche,[1] a force whose mythological image is the devouring aspect of the Great Mother.

Normally, the urge toward growth outweighs the regressive component of the personality. However, pathologies can occur that cause the individual to fear inner development. This outcome, Jung said, results from the regressive component achieving predominance over the psyche's developmental urges. He did not, however, specify what circumstances caused an individual's normal fears to accentuate into a fear of psychological development, nor did he discuss the clinical issues involved.

I first became interested in the fear people have of therapeutic progress when I noticed that the psychological condition of a number of my patients did not improve when there was every expectation that it would. As a matter of fact, it was at the very moment when im-

---

[1] *Symbols of Transformation,* CW 5, par. 456.

provement was most expected, when there had been some important insight or deepening of the therapeutic relationship, that they seemed to get worse. They became depressed and anxiously denied progress or regressed in the face of it.

Further analysis of these individuals indicated a corresponding fear of outer achievement—a pattern that included work inhibitions, a failure to complete tasks, the denigration of positive attributes and accomplishments and an inability to make decisions. I observed that people who fear psychological development sabotage all potential successes including friendships, romances and explicit or implicit contests involving skill, talent, attractiveness or popularity.

For example, in their careers, such people suffer inhibitions that can lead to an inability to work at all—or only at boring positions well below their capabilities. If they do manage to achieve, they tend to lose interest in their work or change jobs. A compliment on how well they look or might have performed elicits a self-minimizing retort that is followed by the declaration of how bad they feel, or a recounting of some foolish error they recently made. Such people have difficulty completing tasks. In school, they do not hand papers in on time, do not prepare adequately for tests or cram furiously at the last minute. In relationships, they tend to change partners frequently because of vague dissatisfactions. While there may be no disturbance in their ability to function sexually, they are often unable to enjoy it.

One of the most common manifestations of the fear of psychological development is an inability to make decisions. We have all known people who try to get others to tell them what to do because they themselves do not want to take responsibility for possible mistakes. A person who fears development, however, is not indecisive because he or she is afraid of a wrong decision. It is the unconscious connection between decisiveness and success that arouses fear.

These people at first appeared to be another example of negative therapeutic reaction, an unconscious hostility which manifests in a desire to frustrate the analyst and do themselves harm. Closer examination, however, suggested that rather than hostility these individuals experienced intense unconscious fear of the analyst. They maintained the unconscious fantasy that the analyst opposed their progress and their external achievements despite evidence to the contrary.

My own self-exploration, discussions with colleagues and supervision of other professionals has led me to believe that there exists in the analyst's unconscious a corresponding identification with the devouring aspect of the Great Mother. This is experienced by the analyst as hostility toward the patient's development, together with an impulse to interfere with the therapeutic progress. Such impulses are usually repressed as the analyst naturally tends to identify with the nourishing aspect of the Great Mother. By way of compensation, this causes the desire to devour to exert its effect unconsciously and all the more strongly.

It is important to embrace and consciously carry the regressive as well as the progressive aspects of the unconscious. Rather than being overcome, the death aspect of the soul, that part of the psyche which opposes development and life, needs to be accepted and explored in both patient and analyst.

The regressive aspect of the unconscious regularly manifests in the analytic situation as a fear of therapeutic progress. In what follows I will describe some of the developmental conflicts and anxieties that undermine analytic progress. My experience has shown that the primary factors involved are separation anxiety, envy and depression. On a low to moderate level these anxieties exist in everyone; they are part of the human condition. However, if traumatically corroborated by the developing individual's environment, these fears become extreme and lead to psychological disorder. In my discussion, I will emphasize the transference-countertransference patterns that each of these anxieties give rise to and suggest an appropriate therapeutic approach.

Separation anxiety

Mahler's observations of mothers with their children indicate that psychological birth does not coincide with biological birth.[2] Immediately after physical birth the child remains merged in a psychological union with the mother. Separation from the mother refers to the child's emergence from this symbiotic fusion. Through the

---

[2] See M. Mahler, F. Pine and A. Bergman, *The Psychological Birth of the Human Infant.*

establishment of a sense of physical separation from the mother, a sense of separateness from the world at large is also established. This self/other differentiation gradually leads to intrapsychic representations of the individual self distinguished from the object world. The process of separation from the mother creates anxiety due to the child's awareness of its helpless and dependent state.

In his mythological studies Erich Neumann came to similar conclusions.[3] The ability to differentiate between subject and object marks the moment human consciousness is born. The development of ego-consciousness and its separation from the unconscious parallels the individual's objective separation from mother, father and family. In archetypal dynamics, the separation of ego-consciousness from the unconscious under the pressures of the progressive urges of the psyche arouses a corresponding reaction from the inertia of the psyche, the instinctual desire to not develop.

Ontogenetically, separation from the biological mother creates anxiety due not only to the child's undeveloped state, but also to the projection of the regressive component of psychic energy onto the mother. The child then fears that the mother does not support growth and separation, and expects a negative reaction such as abandonment when it strives for independence.

Mothers may also experience conflicts over separation due to their own separation anxiety. Such mothers so enjoy their children's dependence that they discourage their groping for independent functioning instead of promoting gradual separation. When the child begins to walk, for instance, rather than giving it a gentle push while providing the security of their emotional availability, they first hold on and then push the child precipitously into premature autonomy.

In extreme cases, some mothers suffer so much separation anxiety they are unable to bear it. When their young children reach the separation stage they find the anxiety intolerable and defensively withdraw. The child, rather than having the secure feeling that mother will always be there, is afraid that if it separates there will be no one to return to. Fearing annihilation, it clings to the mother. This eases the mother's anxiety and she rewards the child with love. Soon the

---

[3] See *The Origins and History of Consciousness,* pp. 102-127.

child comes to feel that any sign of independence, self-assertion or initiative is frightening to the mother and will lead to abandonment, while weakness, clinging or failure will be rewarded.

For example, a woman had suffered consistent abandonment as a child whenever she attempted to separate from her mother and assert her individuality. She recalled that every evening her mother asked her to recount her whole day's experience. One day the child refused, and the mother withdrew in silence. After what seemed like hours, the little girl gave in and told her mother about her day. On another occasion, when she was very young, she had insisted on choosing the clothes she wanted to wear rather than, as was customary, having her mother choose her outfit. At this sign of independence the mother had stalked out of the apartment and left the child alone. During this period the little girl fantasized that her mother would never return and that she would be left to die. She experienced such overwhelming anxiety that when her mother finally returned the little girl begged her to choose her clothes.

This woman was very indecisive and had a history of failing to complete tasks. Ten years before, she had dropped out of college with only one semester to go before graduation. She had returned to college before entering analysis but could not decide on a major. She never got her papers in on time. If she did complete something successfully she became depressed. Her analysis followed a similar pattern. Every advance was followed by a severe depression and regression. Her fantasies and dreams indicated a fear that I really did not want her to grow. Another fear was that I would force her out of analysis prematurely. After passing an examination and feeling seriously depressed instead of proud, she reported the following dream.

> An old woman dressed in black was sitting on a large chair like a throne. Next to her lay a large dog. This woman, who had magical powers, was completely evil. Earlier in the dream I had done something well. In her presence I was afraid and became weak and indecisive. This made her happy. Her chair was made out of material similar to yours [the analyst's].

In archetypal terms, the old woman in the dream is a "terrible mother." She is associated with the goddess Hecate whose accoutrements include dogs, madness and vampires. A death goddess,

Hecate is associated with the regressive aspect of the personality, that part of a person that resists growth.

In ancient times, sacrifices to Hecate were made at crossroads. A common association to the image of crossroads is the need to make a decision, choose a direction. A decision is an act of independence that implies volition to act on one's own. Rather than resolving uncertainty unconsciously, via an identification with parental figures, conscious decision implies separation of the ego from the unconscious, and is thus indicative of psychological development. Given these implications, it is not surprising that decisions arouse separation anxiety.

These reflections on the relationship of decisions to psychological growth help to understand my patient's difficulty. Her associations indicated that choice meant separation from her mother and acceptance of conscious responsibility for herself and her life. While consciously desirable, her exacerbated childhood fears made such signs of inner development intolerable.

The particular conflicts that people with severe separation anxiety experience around the issue of psychological development become active in the analytic relationship. When the patient experiences therapeutic progress, the anxious, withdrawing aspect of the mother image may be projected onto the analyst. The patient may then relate to the projected negative mother image with weakness and failure. The analyst who identifies with the projection may feel separation anxiety and defensively withdraw.

After a number of years of therapy, the woman mentioned above began a session by commenting positively on her recent development. She mentioned a writing class in which she had overcome her fear of being attacked and was able to read her work aloud; she even contemplated a public speaking course, which implied that she would some day have something of value to say to others.

As I listened to her my attention was drawn to the monotonous quality of her voice. I suggested she was afraid to tell me her positive feelings due to fear of my attack. She fell silent, became sleepy and yawned continuously. I began to experience separation anxiety, exemplified by a fantasy that she would leave analysis amidst accusations of my incompetence. On the basis of my countertransference fantasy, I commented that her sleepiness indicated an angry rejection of my intervention; it was not even worth staying awake for. She then expressed her anger: Why had I focused on her voice? That was the negative, regressive aspect of her communication. Why had I not observed and commented on the positive experiences she had described? I then realized and acknowledged that I had identified with and acted out her negative mother who would withdraw and call her "little thing" whenever my patient tried to develop herself.

On the other hand, when the patient becomes aware of psychological growth, the positive feelings of accomplishment may be projected onto the analyst. The patient may then identify with the withdrawing mother and threaten to leave analysis in order to make the analyst feel insecure and needy. The analyst who identifies with the projection of the patient's abandoned ego may feel afraid of losing the patient. This can lead to the analyst's clinging, depression or retaliatory aggression.

A colleague asked me to consult on a case that was causing him difficulty. He had become identified with and was acting out his patient's projection of her withdrawing mother. Whenever the patient felt successful in her personal life or about the progress she was making in analysis, the analyst worried she would no longer need him and would leave analysis. He experienced intense anxiety over this thought. To defend against his fear of separation, the analyst unconsciously withdrew, causing the patient to feel insecure and react by clinging. The analysand experienced the analyst's emotional unavailability as a terrifying threat.

When the analyst became conscious of his behavior, he became frightened of the desire to undermine his patient and overcompensated by encouraging her growth. The patient's dreams and associations indicated that she misunderstood the analyst's excessive encouragement as an attempt to be rid of her. As part of her clinging defense, the patient then asked if a friendship would be possible once the analysis was successfully completed. The analyst's defensive reassurance calmed the analysand, but her dreams showed despair. While she had been consciously reassured, she had unconsciously realized that her anxiety would never be analyzed because she had been implicitly told that separation would never occur.

Envy

Envy, the felt conviction that "anything I need will be withheld from me, so I will spoil or otherwise destroy the withholding object," is one of the most difficult emotions to experience and integrate. A great deal has been written about the role of envy in people's personalities, especially in those with narcissistic problems.[4] Less has been written about the fear of other people's envy and its effect on personal development.

People who suffer excessive fear of envy were commonly raised by a narcissistic parent incapable of positive mirroring. Such parents gain their self-worth and identity through the achievements of their children, whom they experience as extensions of themselves. Since the child exists to mirror the parent, the child must not lay claim to specialness. The child's pride indicates that the positive attributes and achievements belong to the child rather than the parent. This arouses the narcissistic parents' envy. They feel worthless; intense feelings of inferiority are activated by the relationship they assume between someone having something valuable and being valuable.

To prevent the painful feelings of envy and concomitant self-depreciation, narcissistic parents attack what they consider the source of their envy, the child's value. With very primitive parents, this can manifest as a direct, enraged attack, or as a refusal to provide things necessary to enhance the child's attributes. In subtler cases, parents' envy may cause them not to admire their child's attributes or withdraw at their demonstration.

Fear of the narcissistic parents', or one's own, projected envy often leads to conflicted feelings over development. An extremely handsome analysand characterized himself as homely; he remembered that his mother aggressively derided his looks. He was also gifted intellectually; these abilities were also denigrated by his mother, who had not been allowed to attend college by her own parents and felt inferior to her college-educated husband. The mother, in turn, prevented her son from accepting a scholarship. The analysand became afraid of his positive attributes, because he knew they would

---

[4] See, for instance, Ann and Barry Ulanov, *Cinderella and Her Sisters: The Envied and the Envying*.

arouse his mother's envy and lead to aggressive criticism. He responded by depreciating his own abilities and successes.

Like others subject to their mother's envy, the analysand failed to exercise his potential to the fullest. While he did manage to become very successful as an actor, he defended himself against the introjected envious mother by belittling his acting career as stupid and useless work. Finally, at the height of his success, he abruptly quit and went back to college. Again, his intellectual gifts made him successful. But he could not enjoy this either. He chose an academic career he was emotionally unsuited for, worried constantly about grades despite being a straight A student, and made himself generally miserable. Unconsciously, he was placating his mother. Essentially he was saying to her: "Even though I'm doing well at these things there is nothing for you to be envious of because I am miserable and getting no value from any of it."

The relationship with the envious parent is made manifest in the analytic relationship. When the analysand is making progress the envious parent may be projected onto the analyst. In fear of, and defense against, the expected envy, the patient is likely to demean personal accomplishments. The analyst, via identification with the projected envy, might experience envious rage and a desire to spoil the patient's positive feelings. If the analyst acts out the envious reactions, the patient will experience a repetition of the relationship with the envious parent rather than the mirroring necessary to allow the experience of positive attributes and accompanying self-esteem.

A number of years ago, I worked with a young man who was afraid to succeed. His father was narcissistic and would respond with sadistic envy whenever anyone's accomplishments took attention away from him. The father had spoiled all the patient's achievements as a student athlete and later as a professional singer by demeaning comments.

During the first few months of the analysis, the patient, after significant early resistance due to fear of envy, began to develop in areas of his personality in which I was still limited. My own unresolved envy was stimulated by an identification with the patient's projection of his narcissistic father. I imagined that the patient's analysis was better than my own and I envied the patient not only his analysis but the creative therapist who I imagined was the source of the patient's psychological growth; that is, I envied the fact that I could not be analyzed by myself! Rather than mirroring the patient, my envy led me to spoil his therapeutic progress by pointing out what he still had to accomplish.

When I finally became conscious of my envious desire to spoil the analysis I defensively overcompensated and intrusively praised the patient's positive qualities. This overstimulated the patient's grandiosity and aroused his fear of losing contact with reality. In addition, his dreams indicated that he misunderstood my inordinate acclaim to be due to my need to enhance my own self-esteem. He believed that his progress in the analysis was for my benefit, and that his function was to mirror me as he had his envious father.

On the other hand, a patient might identify with the envious parent and envy the analyst's achievements. The patient feels incapable of ever experiencing the real or fantasied self-esteem of the analyst and attempts to make the analyst feel inferior by the use of demeaning comments and behavior. The envious patient may even cause the analysis to fail just so the analyst will not feel successful. If the analyst does not understand this, he or she can become frustrated and resentful. This might eventually culminate in the analyst's actual depression and a defensive attempt to terminate the analysis.

Depression

Research indicates that people who are likely to develop a depressive disorder suffer a severe loss of love early in life and develop the idea that some personal evil was responsible for the loss.[5] This conclusion is usually supported by parental moral criticism emphasizing the child's "badness."

While they despair, however, individuals with depressive pathology harbor the unconscious idea that the other has not been lost irrevocably. The idea that the other can be made loving again is based on the experience that the other once was loving. Spitz observed in a study of infants that those who became depressed had a positive

---

[5] See below, chapt. 7, for an extended discussion of depression.

mothering experience that they lost.[6] Those infants who had never had positive mothering did not develop depression. As a result of this original care, and the idea that childish evil caused its loss, the depressive patient believes that by the proper form of redemptive behavior the other can be made loving again. The unconscious wish is that the redemption of the other will also redeem one's self-esteem.

For such patients, it is critical to avoid a contemporary experience of loss that would arouse the earlier childhood experience. Activities that might result in loss arouse depressive anxiety and are avoided. If a loss of love, actual or fantasied, does occur, they respond with redemptive acts of submission.

People who are seriously depressed are very dependent. They have strong associations, originating in childhood experiences, with loss of love resulting from independence, on the one hand, and to the possibility of regaining love by becoming dependent on the other. Successful behavior is associated with strength and independence which in turn is associated with being unlovable and bad. When they recognize themselves as feeling successful, the childhood complex of loss of love is activated. They automatically respond by trying to turn the projected rejecting parent back into an accepting figure by redemptive, submissive behavior. They become helpless, weak and self-reproachful.

One analysand with a depressive disorder associated her successful career in real estate with the ability to take care of herself. Since, unconsciously, having something done for her meant dependence and love, being successful connoted being unloved and led to a depressive reaction that demeaned the value of her accomplishments. Her self-reproach indicated that she did not love herself and needed the other to take care of her. To assure herself and others that nothing good came from her own functioning, she also attributed her success to others who had played only minor parts in her career.

Depressed individuals suffer excessive and irrational guilt: they feel unworthy of having anything good happen to them. Since psychological development arouses painful feelings of guilt, they become afraid of therapeutic progress.

---

[6] R. Spitz, "Anaclitic Depression: An Inquiry into the Genesis of Psychiatric Conditions in Early Childhood."

The patient mentioned above, for example, responded to her progress in analysis by worsening her condition. In her transference fantasy, I represented her mother who felt inferior and withdrew into depression whenever the analysand felt positive about her abilities. To mitigate her guilt and forestall the feared loss of my love, my patient would try to submit to me via depression. She would become demanding, critical and angry if I failed to respond to her helplessness with advice, control or other caretaking actions. Thus, despite overt encouragement, she felt guilty because, in her fantasy, she caused me to become depressed over her successful growth.

People who are depression-prone frequently grew up in situations demanding that they develop extraversion as a defense against the threat of loss. They were usually reared in households in which the parents forbade the children any modes of understanding other than those directed by the parents. As a consequence, the attention of these individuals became directed almost exclusively toward understanding and satisfying the other. The depression-prone can also develop a fear of introversion. Introspection and the recognition of individual reactions are themselves acts of separateness, independence and selfhood—the very qualities feared because they lead to the threat of loss of love.

The development of an orientation toward others, and fear of their own reactions, cause depressives difficulty in situations that demand choice. To choose, rather than to have a decision presented by an authority, is to be separate, autonomous and independent. These qualities raise the issue of loss of love for nonsubmission. Choice also involves being able to evaluate. Depressive-prone individuals, with their extraverted orientation, look to others to see what they want, and choose what will please someone else in order to receive love. Rather than looking to the situation itself and discriminating with their own thoughts and feelings, they often feel confused in situations of choice and will helplessly appeal to any available authority to tell them what to do.

The depressed woman mentioned above asked the I Ching for a decision. When the answer was unsatisfactory she tried, via her depression, to induce her next authority, the analyst, to make the choice. In the patient's transference fantasy I carried the image of her mother, who wanted her to be weak and helpless. Simply because a situation of choice was presented, the threat of loss of love was also there and she unconsciously reexperienced her original childhood loss. Her depression was both a reaction to her loss and an appeal, through submission, for the analyst/mother to become loving again.

My countertransference reactions included experiencing depressed, rejecting feelings, similar to those the patient ascribed to her mother, whenever my patient began to show signs of therapeutic growth. At such times I actually felt like withdrawing from her. Awareness of my withdrawal aroused feelings of pity for my analysand's suffering and guilt over not being helpful enough. It was often difficult not to defend against my pity and guilt by switching over to an identification with the nourishing aspect of the Great Mother and satisfying my patient's demand for advice and overt support. Experience with this patient, as well as with other depressives, however, has shown me that excessive and inappropriate sympathy and caretaking does not encourage growth, rather it reaffirms the connection between submission and parental love.

Conclusions

In my work with patients who suffer from conflicts which lead to expectations of punishment for psychological development I have found most successful a therapeutic approach in which reductive-causal work precedes "synthesis." Experience has shown me that premature encouragement of the developmental urges of the psyche through synthetic interpretations arouses unconscious fears and their corresponding defenses in the analysand.

Jung was not inimical to reductive analysis—he was opposed only to its dogmatic, exclusive and inappropriate application. As detailed above in chapter one, he suggested that either a reductive or synthetic approach might be appropriate, depending on the particular therapeutic needs of the patient. The reductive approach is called for "when there is something that must be destroyed, dissolved, or reduced."[7] The reductive approach frees psychic energy from pathological mani-

---

[7] "On the Psychology of the Unconscious," *Two Essays on Analytical Psychology,* CW 7, par. 65.

festation by relating the contemporary neurotic behavior to the earlier conflicts from which it derived.

During the reductive phase of psychotherapy people learn to know those unconscious automatic reactions that are hostile to the development of their personality. Reduction helps to establish a conscious relationship between development and the specific childhood fears with which it is associated. Consciousness of these irrational expectations can help free the individual from their power. This part of the work emphasizes the exploration of childhood conditioning through the transference relationship.

Another value of a reductive approach is that it brings out the personal negative transference. This gives the analysand the chance to become conscious of the dark side of the Self. Becoming aware of fear, hurt and rage is a critical developmental experience. Through the transference the patient first fears, then hates, those who, the patient fantasizes, interfere with his or her development.

Misunderstood countertransference reactions can interfere with this process. The analyst has to tolerate being experienced as a non-nurturing, cruel parental figure. In addition, one has to be willing to feel the hostile desire to interfere with the analysand's development. The particular inner reactions of the analyst, whether abandoning, envious or unloving, help to understand the corresponding fears of the analysand. An analyst might become inappropriately supportive in order to reassure the frightened patient that he or she does not feel negative toward the patient's development. Such countertransference reactions prevent negative fantasies from surfacing in the transference. When an analyst demonstrates support too soon, the analysand feels aggression to be inappropriate and so further represses it— along with the energy necessary to support development.

When the regressive fears of development have been resolved, the progressive urges inherent in the psyche resume the process of impelling the growth of the personality. According to Jung, the subsequent maturing is neither haphazard nor a function of conscious decision, but is determined by the need for individuation. A synthetic approach that encourages these developmental tendencies by linking them to the goals symbolized in unconscious products is then necessary.

The synthetic stage is most important for resolving fear of development conflicts on something more than a level of identification with collective goals. One of the things that has become apparent to me is that the fear of psychological development is often related to and symbolic of a fear of individuality. It is the person's very nature and destiny that was really suppressed in childhood. People must recognize that they cannot necessarily be what they consciously decide or have been collectively conditioned to be. To be truly an individual a person must be able to recognize and apply his or her energy toward fulfillment in the direction they are meant to develop. When people overcome their fear of inner development, the fear of achieving outer goals also abates. In many instances, the outer goal itself— whether for fame, position, love or something else, is reexamined and altered when it is realized as inappropriate to the needs of the inner person.

Individuals who are freed from collective identifications are free to experience who they actually are and to choose activities that express their individuality rather than collective norms. Inner experiences and outer activities are then sensed to be a representation of their very nature. As a matter of fact, even everyday activities take on the quality of a religious experience, and one's own self is experienced as a vessel through which manifest one's true creative energies. Only through such experience can life be imbued with meaning.

I'll close with a last example.

Sarah, a twenty-five-year-old student, had started college with the intention of becoming a physician. She was enroled in a pre-med program and was one of the top students. As she approached graduation she became unsure of her career choice and switched over to the study of law. This switch necessitated retaking a number of courses and delayed her graduation for two years. Again Sarah did well, but, as before, became unsure of her career choice as graduation approached. She changed her major for a third time, to teaching. This career choice had previously not been of interest to her. However, she was encouraged to pursue teaching by her father and her boyfriend, who both felt that medicine and law were too masculine and would interfere with Sarah's primary responsibility of motherhood. Her college advisor suggested she seek therapy when she realized this latest career choice was a result of emotional conflict and would not be in Sarah's long term best interests.

Through analysis of the negative transference, Sarah discovered and worked through her childhood fears of rejection by her father, competitive aggression from her brothers, anxieties about being considered deviant for pursuing a "masculine" career in medicine, and finally fears of her mother's envy of Sarah for developing a feminine identity not limited by the traditional ideas her mother had identified with.

But the event that ultimately helped Sarah overcome her regressive fears was her realization of her personal commitment to her own development. It was not becoming a doctor that was really important to Sarah, though that was one form it took, rather it was becoming her own person. This is what her infantile longings were really trying to prevent. And this is what Sarah ultimately stood up for.

From within, a sense of herself as an individual had slowly begun to take shape. This inner sense of self first appeared to Sarah in a dream of an abandoned blond child she was required to nurse and raise. In the dream, Sarah's mother demanded she get rid of the child. At first Sarah complied, hiding the child in the center of a complicated maze. But she realized that without her the child would not survive and, what was also clearly evident, without the child Sarah herself would be incomplete. So Sarah went on a long arduous journey and recovered the child.

When she awoke Sarah immediately realized that the child was her own individuality; that she, like other human beings, had a unique destiny. To stand up for and live that destiny was really the goal she had always feared.

5
Idealization:
A Clinical Discrimination

Admiration occurs when we recognize and value qualities in others that we may not have ourselves. Our perceptions may lead us further into feelings of inferiority or envy but the perceptions are none the less accurate. Idealization, on the other hand, indicates something extreme and unreal. In this case, our perceptions of the other are exaggerated and we may even ascribe to them the coveted qualities of happiness, power, goodness and omnipotence.

Idealization is a normal occurrence in childhood. It manifests itself in the fantasies of omnipotence which children have about their parents. As development proceeds, these feelings are slowly replaced by more realistic perceptions. When this does not occur, and the earliest forms of idealization continue past their age-appropriate phase, idealization becomes pathological.

Jung's Approach to Idealization

Jung, like many psychoanalytic writers,[1] recognized that idealization had both normal and pathological aspects. As a normal developmental phenomenon, he acknowledged that the first objects of idealization were the parents.

However, Jung differed from the psychoanalytic writers in that they viewed the idealized parental images as made up of the actual, though exaggerated, qualities of the real parents. Jung, on the other hand, found the source of the idealization not in the personal experiences of childhood, but in the projection of archetypes.

For Jung, the parents are the recipients of archetypal projections from the child; these projections give the parents their omnipotent

---

[1] See M. Klein, "Some Theoretical Conclusions Regarding the Emotional Life of the Infant"; O. Kernberg, *Borderline Conditions and Pathological Narcissism*, pp. 275-279; H. Kohut, *Restoration of the Self*, pp. 98-101.

72

qualities. He says that these images "outweigh the influence of sensory stimuli and mold them into conformity with a *pre-existing psychic image.*"[2] It is the numinosity of the archetypes that supplies the exaggerated qualities, not the actuality of the parents. A mother becomes an all-good, bountiful mother primarily because the nourishing aspect of the Great Mother is projected, not because the personal mother's nourishing qualities are exaggerated. If development proceeds normally, according to Jung, there occurs an increasing discrimination between the real figures of the parents and the archetypal forms. The archetypal images, and the energy associated with them, fall into the unconscious of the growing personality and are available for future projection.

While most writers agree that idealization is a normal part of childhood development and has a mature form appropriate to adult life, they also recognize a pathological form. Jung accepted this when he said: "Idealization is a hidden apotropaism; one idealizes whenever there is a secret fear to be exorcised."[3]

Since Jung was not primarily interested in the clinical manifestations of idealization, he did not elaborate on its defensive use. When he did have occasion to mention idealization as a clinical phenomenon, he did so primarily to elucidate a transpersonal issue. For example, he described the case of a woman who overvalued him and attributed superhuman qualities to him. He concluded that the overvaluation was a function of an archetypal urge "to free a vision of God from the veils of the personal, so that the transference to the person of the doctor was no more than a misunderstanding on the part of the conscious mind."[4] Jung's clinical approach in this case consisted of explaining his idea to the patient who, he reported, had an intellect able "to appreciate the theoretical possibility of the new hypothesis."[5] Ultimately, the patient's idealization led to the development of a transpersonal control-point.

---

[2] "Concerning the Archetypes and the Anima Concept," *The Archetypes and the Collective Unconscious,* CW 9i, par. 135.

[3] "Psychological Aspects of the Mother Complex," ibid., par. 192.

[4] "The Relations Between the Ego and the Unconscious," *Two Essays on Analytical Psychology,* CW 7, par. 214.

[5] Ibid., par. 216.

Other writers, following Jung, have focused on the transpersonal aspect of idealization.[6] As a consequence, the pathology of idealization remains relatively undiscriminated in Jungian literature. In addition, with the dissemination of Kohut's work, there has been a tendency to associate all manifestations of idealization with narcissistic character disorders. But idealization is present in mature, healthy individuals as well as those who manifest various pathological conditions. Consequently, it is necessary to discriminate normal from pathological idealization. Idealization that follows an unhindered developmental sequence from primitive to mature is normal. Pathological idealization is defensive and fixated. In addition, each form of disordered idealization has its own dynamics and therapeutic necessities.

The aim of this chapter is to discriminate clinically between these disorders, describing various forms of pathological idealization and connecting them to distinct psychological conditions. I emphasize transference and countertransference issues and suggest appropriate analytic responses.

Specific Transference and Countertransference Reactions

Depressive neurosis

A patient with a depressive neurosis idealizes the analyst for two significant reasons. The primary motivation is to defend against feelings of aggression toward the analyst. A secondary reason is that association with a valuable other mitigates the patient's feelings of worthlessness.

The depressive represses anger and other feelings that imply independence or initiative and in their stead substitutes submissive behavior.[7] Both the repression and the submission alleviate anxious feelings about abandonment and allow for the hope of regaining the love experienced at an earlier age. When an analysand senses angry feel-

---

6 See E.F. Edinger, *Ego and Archetype,* p. 68; M. Jacoby, *The Analytic Encounter,* p. 53; N. Schwartz-Salant, *Narcissism and Character Transformation,* p. 43; J. Satinover, "The Mirror of Doctor Faustus: The Decline of Art in the Pursuit of Eternal Adolescence."

7 See below, chapt. 7, for a fuller discussion of these issues.

ings toward the analyst, usually for not giving adequate care or allowing enough dependency, the patient fears that the analyst will withdraw love. In fantasy, the depressive always hopes to gain more love; all he or she needs to do is find the proper form of submission. Then a reaction formation occurs: an unacceptable feeling is converted into its opposite and the ego experiences this opposite feeling. Rather than anger and contempt, the patient experiences idealizing feelings that are accompanied by depression and inferiority.

A woman had been suffering from a serious depression for two months. It began after a dance class when an authoritarian teacher commented favorably on her work and asked her to say what was positive about herself and her performance. This opportunity to give herself gratification and value constellated a childhood pattern of loss of love. The woman's mother had rejected her whenever the analysand was happy, excited, looking forward to something or feeling proud of herself, and the mother could not take any credit for the situation. This continued into adulthood. Whenever the patient felt responsible for her own good feelings she became depressed because they were immediately, but unconsciously, followed by fear of loss of love.

This patient was, as are most depressives, very well behaved. She always paid her bills promptly. That month, however, she not only did not pay her therapy bill on time, she forgot her check for the next two sessions. The second session after her bill was due she was exceedingly depressed and informed me of the again forgotten check. She then related the following dream: "I had an appointment with a new therapist for one session. I arrived early and she told me to wait in a silo nearby and draw pictures of the rats that lived there. I told her I was allergic to rats and did not want to do it." Her associations indicated that the new therapist was an omnipotent figure who would only require one session to solve her problems. The rats represented her "disgusting" negative feelings.

I suggested that she was angry at me for not solving the problem of her depression more decisively and quickly—more omnipotently —and that forgetting payment was an expression of her anger. She vehemently denied this and instead told me how helpful, giving, smart, supportive and generous I had been over the years, and especially during the recent depressive crisis. She had forgotten to pay me because she was bad and stupid and always ruined everything. She continued with further self-reproach.

Countertransference reactions to being idealized, combined with the patient's self-hate, often lead an analyst to take a supportive, caretaking position. The analyst points out that everyone makes mistakes, that the patient should not be so self-critical, that the patient has many good points and so on, rationalizing that such support counters the patient's sadistic superego. What is really happening, however, is that the analyst is reinforcing the patient's submissive behavior. In the patient's unconscious, the punishing, rejecting parents have been intrapsychically aroused and projected onto the analyst. Faced with the threat of loss of love for angry feelings, the patient represses the anger and unconsciously converts it into an idealization through defensive reaction formation. The interpersonal threat that arises from the projected parental figures is warded off by further overt idealization of the analyst and depressive self-reproaches that arouse the analyst's pity.

In the example given, I was able to contain my countertransference guilt and pity and continue to gently but firmly point out to my patient that she was showing every indication of being angry, but, because of fear, was repressing the anger and behaving submissively. Eventually, her angry feelings emerged. She had been depressed for months; if I were competent, I would have already pulled her out. Not only was she financially burdened with my fees, she was paying for incompetence! Another issue was that I had allowed another patient to attack her in group therapy. This induced the fantasy that I favored the other patient in the same way as her mother had favored a sibling. She hated me for this. After expressing these feelings she became quite frightened and even more depressed.

It is important to note that expressing her aggressive feelings had only a temporary alleviative effect on the depression. What finally did help was when she became fully conscious that the aggressive feelings she had expressed made her fear losing my approval, that the fantasied loss made her depressed and that her depression was also a form of submission to win me back.

Again, however, after realizing all of this, the patient became even more deeply depressed. Over the next few weeks, we discovered that this depression was related to the sacrifice of her relationship to the Self in an attempt to obtain love. The following material emerged:

A number of weeks earlier, as a result of a minor accident, I had worn a brace on my arm to a group therapy session. During this session the patient fantasized that I was angry at myself over the injury. My display of anger at myself (in her fantasy) was an admission of error and a sign of weakness. I was no longer ideal.

As an idealized person, my love and acceptance could mitigate her feelings of being unlovable. She had developed a bargain relationship with me similar to the one she had had with her mother. Following this earlier pattern, she attempted to determine my ideal of her and then make herself into that in return for my approval. What now depressed her was that I no longer had the idealized qualities for which she had made so many painful sacrifices. If I was no longer ideal, then the attainment of my approval would no longer mitigate her self-hate. She had sacrificed her soul for nothing. Her depression was related to this deep sense of losing contact with the Self.

Borderline condition

In *The Origins and History of Consciousness,* Erich Neumann says that during its early stages of development, the ego has not yet unified into a cohesive psychological structure.[8] Similarly, the image of the Great Mother is not unified. Instead, the nourishing and devouring polarities of this image are experienced sequentially. Normally, as development proceeds, the ego develops into a cohesive structure that experiences the polarities of the Great Mother as part of a unified archetypal image.

The archetypal process whereby ego and object images are integrated manifests in personal development when introjections and identifications are synthesized into stable psychic structures. At first introjections and identifications are built up separately and experienced as good or bad, depending on whether they were associated with love or aggression. As development proceeds, the idealized all-good object images are integrated with the all-bad object images, and

---

[8] "The Creation Myth: The Great Mother," pp. 39-101.

the same holds true for good and bad self images. This integration leads to realistic object and self images.

Because of excessive anxiety and other traumas, this process fails in people who develop borderline disorders. In archetypal terms, the nourishing, all-good aspect of the Great Mother is forcibly kept apart from the devouring, all-bad aspect. The ego, too, does not develop into a unified structure.

While the division into good and bad happens originally due to the lack of integrative capacity of the ego, it is later used defensively by the borderline person to prevent anxiety and to protect the ego core built around positive introjections. This defensive division of the ego is accomplished through the mechanism of splitting.

Splitting refers to the active process of keeping apart introjections and identifications of opposite quality, such as those determined by love and aggression. Under these pathological circumstances, contradictory ego states are alternately activated; anxiety is prevented since they are kept separate. Splitting usually occurs in combination with other primitive defense mechanisms, such as projective identification, denial and idealization.

The experience of the borderline differs from that of the depressive in that the aggression of the borderline is not experienced as emanating from oneself; instead, one fantasizes that another person is the aggressor. Similarly, in the transference of the borderline person, aggressive and loving feelings for the analyst are split; they are not experienced as directed toward the same person. The feelings exist side by side without affecting each other.

The split-off aggressive feelings are first aroused by frustration and become exaggerated by the normal extremes of infantile emotionality. Then, the aggressive feelings themselves give rise to fears of annihilation and are quickly ejected from the system via projection onto the analyst. The final step for the borderline person is to deny, by means of idealization, the analyst's hostility and the borderline's own fears. The patient therefore makes the analyst into an exaggerated all-good figure to defend against the analyst's badness.

The borderline's compartmentalization of people into all-good and all-bad, with the concomitant possibility of complete, abrupt shifts from one extreme to the other, makes the transference contradictory and confusing. As a beginner to the field of psychotherapy, I was often surprised and disappointed when, after establishing what seemed to be a close relationship with a patient—which I later realized was based on my failure to differentiate between intimacy and idealization—I would find a message on my answering machine that the patient was dropping out of treatment.

If I called the patient to discuss the issue, or to at least terminate the analysis in a more personal manner, I would be met by a refusal to talk or a cold explanation of how the analysis was not helping. Pointing out that just last week the person had mentioned the value of the treatment would elicit either a bland denial or some vague recollection that had no emotional relevance.

In addition to the transference being contradictory, the countertransference reaction, especially where the analyst's self-esteem is involved, is also subject to abrupt shifts from positive to negative.

One man with a borderline disorder began a session by commenting on his recently acquired ability to feel close to me and intimate with his wife. Meanwhile, compulsive fears that his wife was having an affair with a neighbor had diminished. He attributed these positive developments to me and the therapy and expressed gratitude at his good fortune in working with someone so skilled. I felt great pride in having been able to help a person with such difficult and long-standing problems, especially after so many of his previous attempts at therapy had failed.

As I listened to him I was struck by the affectless quality of his voice. I drew this to his attention, without commenting on what he was saying. During the ensuing silence I began to experience persecutory anxiety, exemplified by an abandonment fantasy that the patient would leave the analysis without saying another word to me. I was amazed at the sudden change in my self-esteem; in a flash I had gone from excessive pride and confidence to feeling incompetent! I realized that my observation must have angered the patient and caused him to shift me from the all-good to the all-bad compartment, and that I was experiencing that shift through my countertransference fantasy. I suggested that his silence indicated an angry rejection.

My patient then expressed his anger and hurt: The experience of intimacy was new and tenuous for him, and my focus on the inadequacy of his expression had caused him to doubt his accomplishment. From pride in himself he had abruptly shifted into feelings of hopelessness and despair. Similarly, he had begun to experience me as a threatening and dangerous person looking for opportunities to attack. He had completely forgotten that he had started the session with feelings of intimacy and trust toward me.

One of the difficulties in progressing analytically with borderline patients is that their defenses render them unconscious of anxiety. Thus one of the prime motivations for analytic work, the relief of anxiety, is absent. A preliminary goal in working with analysands of this type is to make them conscious of their anxiety. Another difficulty is that when people split into good and bad, they are unable to experience ambivalence. A major goal in the therapy of such people is therefore to synthesize the split in their egos and inner images so that they can experience ambivalence.

Technically, in the case of borderline patients, interpretations oscillate between reduction and synthesis. In the area of idealization, for example, the idealizing defense is first interpreted reductively. This brings to the patient's consciousness the fear of the analyst's hostility. Only after confronting this fear can the patient be made aware that the fantasized hostility is really an expression of his or her own aggression. These interpretations will create paranoid anxiety in the patient. The aggression and the idealization must then be linked in a synthetic interpretation and shown to belong to the patient. An example will illustrate these points.

One day, out of confusion, I started and ended a number of sessions ten minutes early. When I realized the error, I explained my mistake to the affected patients and offered to make up the lost time. One patient who suffered from a borderline-type condition was very upset. His reaction was not due to any feeling of personal slight, but rather to the fact that I had made an error. This broke his idealized fantasy of me as an omnipotent parent who would take perfect care of him. He experienced intense anxiety and his associations were paranoid. Now that I was no longer perfectly good, he felt endangered by me. In his fantasy I was maliciously attempting to make him dependent and vulnerable so that I could vent my sadism on him. I suggested that he kept his paranoid feelings at bay by projecting idealizing qualities onto me. My error had temporarily destroyed the idealizing defense and let loose a flood of paranoid feelings. This comment held together his split image of me. Rather than seeing me as being all-good or all-bad, he could see me as having positive and negative qualities, and thus his feelings about me became ambivalent. Awareness of this lessened his anxiety.

Over the years since this incident, as this patient has begun to experience his own hostile feelings, there has been a marked decrease in his defensive idealizing tendencies and accompanying paranoia.

In contrast to the anger, pity and guilt felt in working with the depressed patient, idealization from borderline patients arouses in the analyst aggressive impulses that are intense and compulsive. Countertransference aggression is often due to identifying with the patient's split-off rage or aggressive behavior which tends to provoke in the analyst a desire to retaliate. I sometimes feel as if these patients were pushing their aggressive feelings into me and as if my countertransference represented the emergence of that part of the patient from my own psyche. I often only discover I have defended against these difficult reactions when I realize I have dissociated and missed long sections of the session. I have learned that when I "space out" and find it difficult to pay attention, I am either defending against the patient's rage that I have introjected, or am identifying with the patient's fear of the rage projected into me.

An even more dangerous response is acting out the driven quality of the sadism and attacking the patient verbally. The analyst needs to be aware that the sadism he or she is experiencing is a countertransference identification with the patient's projected hostility. The analyst's fear of sadistic impulses toward the patient correlate with the patient's fear of being annihilated. Only when the analyst is aware of his or her own sadism and fear can the process of interpreting the patient's fear of the analyst's hostility begin.

Narcissistic character disorder

In the narcissistic character disorder, idealization appears as a defense against envy-related hostile affects and as a result of a fixation in development. Nathan Schwartz-Salant correctly points out that adequate interpretation of the defensive form of idealization leads to the appearance of the developmentally fixated form.[9] The change from defensive to developmentally fixated is indicated by the appearance of the stable idealizing transference.

As a defense against envy, idealization manifests itself in a variety of ways. In one instance the analysand actually idealizes the analyst in order to defend against his or her own envy. A variation is that the envy is projected onto the analyst and the analysand idealizes the analyst to defend against the latter's envy. In another form the patient resists idealizing the analyst in order to avoid the experience of envy that the patient unconsciously knows will occur as a result. In all of these instances the underlying motivations for the defense are painful feelings of intense shame, emptiness, rage and fragmentation of a precarious self.

Therapeutically, the idealizing defense must be interpreted. The interpretation needs to refer to the defended envy and the painful affect that makes the envy so unacceptable. While full reconstruction is seldom necessary, reference to an expected lack of empathic acceptance from the analyst, reminiscent of earlier failures from the parents, is often helpful. If these interpretations are done consistently and empathically, the transference will change from being defensive to being developmentally fixated. The analyst will know the difference by alterations in the countertransference. In the defensive form of idealization, the analyst will feel discord between the overt idealization and the hostile envy that resides behind it. When the analysand resists the idealization in order to defend against his or her own envy, indications of the hidden idealization will appear. In either case, the analyst will not feel an overabundance of self-esteem.

There is a dramatic difference in the countertransference that occurs in response to the developmentally fixated idealizing transference. The analyst will feel elevated beyond the normal feeling of pride in oneself for a job well done. Instead there may occur fantasies of being the best analyst and the only one who could help that particular analysand. At times there may even occur the sensation of floating a few inches above the ground.

The intensity of such fantasies and their occurrence early in the

---

[9] *Narcissism and Character Transformation,* p. 107.

analysis often indicate the possibility of a serious narcissistic character disorder.

In depressive neurosis and borderline conditions idealization is a transient feature of the transference. In the narcissistic character disorder, however, idealization assumes central significance because it reactivates the blocked narcissistic development at the point where the fixation occurred. The analysand maintains self-esteem through merger with the idealized analyst. The refusal or inability of the analyst to accept the idealization threatens the analysand with a serious loss. The analysand often responds to such an empathic failure with an angry insistence that the analyst is as omnipotent as the analysand fantasizes.

The demands on the analyst can become quite confusing and at times the analyst cannot help but disappoint the analysand. The following example will indicate the complexity of the demands idealization places on the analyst.

During a session my office became hot and stuffy and I opened a window. The analysand became enraged and said now there was a draft. Then he claimed that I had purposely tried to make him angry by not paying attention to him. I responded that my behavior was not premeditated and that I had only opened the window to cool off the room. This made him even angrier. He said that despite his original anger, he had really been pleased that I was so in control that I could plan to frustrate and enrage him. If my action was not premeditated, then his idealization of me was shattered. Even though he had been angry about feeling manipulated, he was proud to be associated with someone who could manipulate him so well.

In contrast to what is required with a defensive idealization, reduction and content interpretation are inappropriate analytic responses to developmentally fixated idealization. Kohut says that the appropriate response to idealization in the narcissistic character disorder is to accept it without interpretation.[10] Interpretations are directed only toward resistances to the idealization's occurrence. After it is established, interpretations are directed toward disruptions in the idealization due to failures of analytic empathy.

---

[10] *Restoration of the Self,* p. 30.

General Countertransference Reactions

The most common reason for difficulty in accepting a patient's idealization is inadequate experience. The analyst has not learned to differentiate a social response from an analytic response. A direct compliment or open admiration often creates inner tensions in the analyst that are alleviated by humility or a compliment in return. Analytically, however, this is incorrect, especially with the narcissistic character disorders. In analytic situations an idealization needs to be either quietly accepted or interpreted in a manner consistent with clinical circumstances.

A second reason for failing to accept the patient's idealization is the analyst's countertransference reactions. An idealization may release narcissistic tensions in the psyche of the analyst. The analyst is filled with grandiose fantasies and feels an exhibitionist desire for more admiration. If the analyst is afraid of this happening, he or she may try to inhibit the patient's attempts at idealization.

Once, during supervision, an analyst-in-training presented a case in which the patient was obviously attempting to idealize her. Whenever the patient presented idealizing fantasies, the analyst responded with a reality statement. The analyst's reasoning was that the patient's tenuous hold on reality necessitated constant differentiation of unconscious fantasies from objective reality. She also reluctantly admitted that she felt hostility at these moments and thought the patient to be needy, weak and wimpish.

Even after it became clear that the patient suffered from a narcissistic character disorder that required idealization for healing, the analyst was still unable to allow it. In discussing her associations to being idealized, she remembered that her mother had been a grandiose woman. The mother had suffered a heart attack and, in her omnipotent way, prematurely returned to work against the doctor's advice. The mother then suffered another major coronary and died. In the analyst's unconscious resided the fear that the patient's idealization would cause her to become like her mother, with consequent loss of reality and self-destructive behavior. After realizing this, the analyst was able to accept the idealization.

There are other instances in which the analyst refuses to analyze defensive idealization. The analyst may be unable to tell the difference between a defensive idealization that needs to be analyzed and idealization that is integral to the developmental process. Countertransference issues can prevent the analyst from making these discriminations.

An analyst may also be unwilling to analyze idealization because it satisfies personal narcissistic needs. He or she needs to be seen as a valuable, wise, good and important person. Often the analyst will rationalize that the defensive idealization is really a developmental idealization and should not be interpreted. In more serious situations the analyst will identify with the patient's fantasy and believe it is an accurate appraisal. Jung noted this danger when he wrote: "The emotions of patients are . . . very contagious when the contents which the patient projects into the analyst are identical with the analyst's own unconscious contents."[11]

Fear of the negative transference is another common reason for the analyst's failure to discriminate and interpret defensive idealization. In most instances a patient's individuation process will require a deep experience of the dark side of the Self. Experientially, this occurs in the analysis via the negative transference. The hurt, rage and hate that are part of the negative transference are a critical developmental experience for the analysand, but it is unpleasant to be the recipient of intense negative emotions. This is especially true when they are directed toward very real weaknesses in the analyst. Even if the hostility is recognized as transferential, it can constellate a painful feeling of inadequacy.

The analyst who has difficulty in accepting personal inadequacies, or has tendencies toward depression or self-hate, may feel threatened by the patient's hostility and try to avoid it by not interpreting the defensive idealization. The analyst may even maintain or reinforce the idealization, unconsciously communicating to the patient that the aggression is too frightening and dangerous. This fosters a split in the analysand. Positive feelings are then reserved for the analyst and negative feelings for the extra-analytic environment. As a consequence, the world outside the analysis remains insidiously hostile.

---

11. "The Tavistock Lectures," *The Symbolic Life,* CW 18, par. 322.

Analysts may also be afraid of the hostility aroused in them by the negative transference. When the patient demeans the analyst and even supportive comments are rejected with contemptuous remarks, the analyst's need to feel competent is frustrated. This narcissistic wound may arouse the analyst's rage. An analyst frightened by his or her own sadistic fantasies will not be able to process this rage or understand it in terms of the transference-countertransference dynamic. In such cases, avoiding the negative transference results in a failure to interpret the defensive idealization.

Conclusions

Jung suggested that idealization serves a purposive religious function for the psyche. As such, it has a teleological significance for the individuation process. Through projection, it offers an opportunity to consciously integrate archetypal images and the energy associated with them.

The issues raised by Jung's hypothesis are complex. For example, it has been shown that idealization manifests in distinct ways in pathologies associated with different developmental issues. How is this to be reconciled with Jung's idea that idealization represents the urge of the Self or God-image to manifest in consciousness? To say that idealization is a projection of archetypal images and energy is not an adequate explanation. A theory of development is necessary to account for both the normal transformations of the idealizing process and its pathological manifestations. I shall offer a few theoretical speculations.

The process of individuation can be understood as the continuous development of the individual toward a unique approximation of the Self, which occurs when the meaning of its energies are embodied in a person's life. This leads to the incarnation of the Self in the phenomenal world.

Idealization is the process through which the numinous aspect of this process is expressed. Out of the merged condition of child and Self comes the projection of the Self onto the parents. Later, the child merges again with the Self through the now idealized parents. As the child develops it experiences the parents more realistically, especially after being disappointed a number of times. The idealization, with its numinosity, is withdrawn and the merger of the Self with the parents gradually ends. In fact, a dual separation occurs. The Self separates from the parents, and the ego loses the connection it formerly maintained with the Self through its merger with the parents. The numinous energy of the withdrawn idealization is internalized and builds up psychic structures that are functional incarnations of the Self.

Kalsched, in reference to the narcissistic character disorder, comes to similar theoretical conclusions.[12] He says that the therapist, through the idealizing transference, embodies for the patient psychological functions such as the regulation of self-esteem. In addition, he suggests that the Self, through idealization, is transmuted into psyche. Schwartz-Salant, also discussing narcissistic character disorders, agrees that the Self unfolds through the development of psychic structures.[13] Unfortunately, both writers arrive at this conclusion through the analysis of mythology. Neither offers significant empirical support for their hypotheses.

When development is inhibited, either through fixation or defense, the individual ceases to evolve in relation to the Self. As a consequence, the numinous energy of the archetypes is not incarnated as psychic structure and the various pathologies of idealization result. From a Jungian point of view, psychopathology is viewed symbolically as well as symptomatically. As a symptom, idealization involves the attribution of miraculous, omnipotent powers to another person. Looked at symbolically, however, the God-like qualities attributed to the other can be understood as expressions of the Self whose incarnation through the development of psychic structure has been frustrated. The symptom becomes a misunderstood symbol. What form the symptom/symbol takes depends on the developmental stage at which the individuation process was restricted.

The ideas presented in this chapter allow for the derivation of clinical theory. In regard to the depressive, I suggest the following.

Idealization has been interpreted as a defense against hostility or as a mitigation of worthless feelings. This is reductive, but it is often

---

12 "Narcissism and the Search for Interiority."
13 *Narcissism and Character Transformation,* p. 43.

necessary to interpret reductively in order to interfere with the depressive's pathological defensive process. Reductive interpretations allow the energy and content behind the defense—for example, repressed aggression and the various dynamics that result in the defense of idealization—to enter consciousness. Without the need to defend against this aggression, a healthier, less conflicted relationship will exist both intra- and inter-psychically. Individuation is advanced via integration of the dark side of the Self.

In addition, reductive interpretation frees the specific energy of the idealization from its pathological manifestation. This energy may then proceed along its normal developmental course. As Kohut has observed, when idealization is allowed to develop normally, it is employed in the development of the psychic structures that regulate self-esteem, results in a stable sense of self and leads to internalized ideals and values. If these psychic structures can be shown to be functional incarnations of the Self, then a step will have been taken in the integration of Jung's ideas with much current clinical information.

6
Masculine Identity Conflicts

The universal energies that manifest in human behavior and attitudes are generally divided into two opposing categories. The Chinese denoted them by the terms Yin and Yang. Another set of terms, coined by the social scientist Parsons, is expressive and instrumental.[1]

Empathy and nurturance are examples of the expressive, or Yin, dimension. Keeping intact the internal affairs of the family by coping with its stresses and strains, the maintenance of smooth relations between family members, giving emotional support and operating as a mediator are all expressive functions. The instrumental, or Yang, position, on the other hand, is competence-directed and goal-oriented, concerned with adaptation to, and communication with, the world outside the family. The instrumental function involves authority, discipline and sound judgment.

One common way society has of differentiating the expressive and instrumental functions is along gender lines, loading male roles heavily, but not exclusively, with the instrumental function and female roles with the expressive function.

For years, American society has considered masculinity to be the mark of the psychologically healthy male and femininity to be the mark of the psychologically healthy female. Recently, however, it has begun to be argued that our current system of gender role differentiation has long since outlived its usefulness, and that it now serves only to prevent both men and women from developing as full human beings. Supporters of this position insist that people should no longer be socialized to conform to outdated standards of gender identity, but should be encouraged to be "androgynous," that is, develop in themselves both the masculine and the feminine, the instrumental and the expressive, Yin and Yang.

A person who is highly identified with a gender role is motivated to maintain a self-image as masculine or feminine, a goal which is

---

[1] T. Parsons and R.F. Bales, *Family, Socialization, and Interaction Process.*

accomplished by not developing, or suppressing, any behavior that might be considered undesirable or inappropriate for his or her sex. Thus, each gender role represents not only the endorsement of "appropriate" attributes, but the simultaneous rejection of qualities commonly associated with the opposite gender role.

In contrast, an androgynous sex role represents the equal endorsement of both masculine and feminine characteristics. The androgynous individual is able to remain sensitive to the changing constraints of a situation and engage in whatever behavior seems most effective at the moment.

Gender roles not only define how men and women consciously identify their egos, they also help determine their unconscious contrasexual natures, their anima or animus. Some people believe that the psychological qualities typically represented by the anima are part of a feminine principle inherently inferior in men, and that the animus represents a masculine principle intrinsically alien to women. I do not agree. Rather, I consider them to be archetypes representing what is undeveloped in an individual's psyche; they symbolize a vast potential, the possibility of becoming.

What causes the potential represented by the contrasexual archetypes not to develop and become integrated into the conscious personality? A primary reason is the tendency for certain behaviors, feelings and attitudes to be dispersed by culture into masculine and feminine roles. By and large, those characteristics considered feminine do not get developed by men, in inverse proportion to the rigidity of a man's gender identification; and vice versa with women.

For example, needs and their satisfaction are considered part of the expressive function, Yin. How an individual deals with needs is really quite complex. One can recognize and satisfy needs through self-reliant behavior or by asking someone else for help, that is, by being dependent. On the other hand, one can be unconscious of needs or aware only of a vague undifferentiated longing. Men are often in this position. Neediness is excluded from the male gender role of self-sufficiency. As a consequence, many men consider dependent feelings to be a sign of weakness and do not develop a conscious relationship to them. Being unconscious and undeveloped, the issue of needs is then associated with the anima. Since what is unconscious is discovered via projection, women and children become the carriers of needs and dependency feelings.

Such men relate to their needs in an undifferentiated or childish way, either not recognizing them at all or being too humiliated to state them and ask for their satisfaction. Like a child that still functions on the basis of *participation mystique,* unconscious identity with others, they expect the women in their lives to read their minds and satisfy their needs. Their feelings are hurt and they pout if this does not happen because they think it means their women really do not love them. This often leads to rage, which they also cannot admit because that would necessitate recognizing that they have been hurt and are needy, something real men do not do.

Jungian psychology has in theory taken the position that psychological androgyny is the path toward wholeness, but in practice there is still a tendency to attribute certain aptitudes, behaviors and feelings to the masculine principle and others to the feminine principle. While it is argued that these principles are archetypal and not related to gender, they have in fact become contaminated by cultural biases.

For instance, despite the fact that typology is supposed to be gender neutral, the functions of thinking and sensation have become associated not just to the archetypal masculine but to the male gender, just as feeling and intuition have become associated with women. One of the unfortunate consequences of such stereotypical gender roles is that the ability to think becomes a male prerogative and to be able to feel becomes female.

When a woman associates Logos with the masculine, her ability to think analytically remains undeveloped. It is undeveloped thinking that is referred to when it is said that women do not think but express animus opinions, or that a woman's animus functions like an inferior man. Such comments are often pejorative, implying that women cannot or should not think, or that thinking is an intrinsically masculine aptitude that a woman discovers through a relationship with her animus. By extension, a woman who can think and enjoys ideas is accused of being too masculine, with the added implication that she is somehow inadequate as a woman.

On the other hand, having a deep, well-differentiated affective life is an expressive function, Yin, and since it is associated with the feminine gender role it is labeled unmasculine. Insofar as a man considers having a deep affective life to be feminine, his affect will exist only as undeveloped potential associated with the anima and will manifest in an inferior way, for instance as moodiness.

Are Logos, self-assertion and independence really masculine? Are Eros, relatedness and nurturance really feminine? I doubt it. These are gender biases. A woman is capable of developing her thinking to be the equivalent of a man's, and a man can differentiate his needs or his feelings as well as a woman. We should not be too quick to assume inherent biological or archetypal differences between men and women without being aware of the serious complications inherent in such opinions.

Let us take aggression as an example. Hormonal research suggests a stronger biological predisposition toward aggressiveness in males than in females. For instance, one study showed that male hormone treatment of pregnant primates increased the incidence of rough-and-tumble play among their female offspring; in humans, girls whose mothers were treated with male hormones while they were pregnant were later more vigorously active and more tomboyish than other girls.[2]

However, females also have male hormones and males have female hormones, the distribution of which varies widely. In addition, family and society tend to reinforce aggressive traits in males and not in females. Our society, for instance, provides numerous blatant role prescriptions of aggressiveness for males, the most obvious being combat service in the military, the different toys boys and girls are given to play with and the male heroes in novels, on TV, and in films who are usually extremely violent. In contrast, our culture reinforces females in nurturance, dependence, obedience and home-centered activities, while it discourages aggression that would be tolerated in males.

Thus, while biology is involved in producing generally greater aggression in men, how and whether this aggression will be expressed is largely effected by personal and cultural history. Parents can interact with a boy in a way that will inhibit his aggression or

---

[2] J. Money and A.A. Ehrhardt, "Prenatal Hormonal Exposure: Possible Effects on Behavior in Man."

with a girl in a way that will enhance hers. Some societies, such as the Tchambuli of New Guinea, even produce relatively aggressive women and passive men.[3]

Does this mean there are no difference between men and women, merely culturally defined gender roles? I do not believe that to be the case either. While the energies which manifest are universal, I suggest that the experience of them differs due to the fact that men and women are biologically different. While a man's biology does not necessarily make him assertive and a woman's does not necessarily make her receptive, their respective anatomies do give them a particular experience of the aggressive and the receptive. I do not believe that men will ever understand the experience of being penetrated in the same way as will a woman. Similarly, the quantity of androgen that the male fetal brain is bathed in will give a man a qualitatively different experience of aggression than a woman. But the abilities to be aggressive, penetrated, related, independent, passive and autonomous are human and common to both.

I'm now going to deal exclusively with masculine psychology.

While siblings, peers and other adults can be quite influential in the development of a child's gender role, the most significant figure for a boy is his father. Whether he is secure or defensive in his gender role will be mostly determined by who his father is and the quality of their relationship. Except in cases of an absent father, the mother is far less important than the father when it comes to the development of a boy's masculine gender role.[4]

The son's identification with his father's masculinity can be either developmental or defensive.

The basis for developmental identification is a nurturing parent-child relationship which motivates the child to reproduce bits of the beloved parent. Defensive identification, on the other hand, is not based on love and affection, but is synonymous with identification with the aggressor. It is a way of reducing anxiety by becoming like the person one is afraid of.

---

[3] M. Mead, *Male and Female,* pp. 114-115.

[4] E.M. Hetherington, M. Cox and R. Cox, "Family Interaction and the Social, Emotional and Cognitive Development of Children Following Divorce."

Research indicates that whether a male's masculinity is based on defensive or developmental identifications is related to paternal nurturance and paternal participation in limit setting and decision making.[5] Paternal nurturance refers to the father's affectionate, attentive encouragement of his child. Paternal nurturance leads to developmental identification; the boy wants to be like the father he loves and who loves and supports him. Similarly, the son's perception of his father's authority, through the father's participation in family decisions and the setting of limits, leads to a developmental identification with a powerful and valued figure.

Taken separately, no one of these factors seems sufficient to ensure that a boy will become masculine. A boy could have a masculine father who is not very involved with his family; or the father could be nurturing but not a very effective or competent model; or he could be very masculine and set limits but not have developed a basic affectionate relationship with his son. All three are necessary.[6]

Men who develop an insecure or defensive masculinity, on the other hand, often grow up in situations with a nonnurturing father who is either passive or dominating.

One study found that adolescent boys low in masculine interest often came from homes in which the father played a traditionally feminine role.[7] The fathers took over activities such as cooking and household chores and generally did not participate in family decision making or limit setting. What seemed to inhibit the boys' masculine development was not their fathers' participation in traditionally feminine activities per se, but their general passivity in family interactions and decision making.

Children who are deprived of a masculine paternal presence are more likely to take a defensive posture of rigid adherence to cultural

---

[5] W.C. Bronson, "Dimensions of Ego and Infantile Identification," pp. 532-545; P.S. Sears, "Child Rearing Factors Related to Playing of Sex-Typed Roles," p. 431; E.M. Hetherington, "A Developmental Study of the Effects of Sex of the Dominant Parent on Sex-Role Preference, Identification, and Imitation in Children," pp. 188-194.

[6] A. Bandura and R.H. Walters, *Adolescent Aggression: A Study of the Influence of Child-Rearing Practices and Family Interrelationships.*

[7] U. Bronfenbrenner, "The Study of Identification Through Interpersonal Perception."

role standards or to avoid expected gender-related behaviors. One study of paternally deprived boys on projective tests and interviews with their mothers indicated that father separation was associated with compensatory masculinity—the boys at times behaving in an exaggerated masculine manner, at other times behaving in a highly feminine manner. The father-separated boys seemed much less secure in their masculinity.[8]

However, it should not be implied from this research that masculinity is founded on an image of male dominance. Research shows that if the father is controlling and restrictive of his son by punishing the son's disagreement with him, the boys are low in masculinity.[9] Extreme paternal dominance of the son squelches the development of independence and competence.

When a boy has a loving relationship with a masculine, competent and nurturing father, he develops the father's masculine characteristics, and, insofar as the father is representative of his culture, the boy develops the behavior and attitudes appropriate for a male. He identifies with traditional masculinity and feels good about his maleness. It is only from this position of masculine security that he can also open himself to the possibility of androgyny.

Research indicates that the relationship between the parents has a large effect on how open the boy is to relating to the inner and outer feminine and his evaluation of the feminine.[10] The quality of communication, respect and cooperation between father and mother has a strong effect on the boy's developing conceptions of male-female relationships and the overall quality of his sex-role functioning. However, while the mother's femininity is important in determining the boy's attitude toward the feminine, that evaluation will occur mostly through the identification with the father and the father's relationship to the mother.

In situations where fathers dominate and devalue their wives, or

---

[8] D.B. Lynn and W.L. Sawrey, "The Effects of Father-Absence on Norwegian Boys and Girls," pp. 258-262; R. Burton, "Cross-Sex Identity in Barbados," pp. 365-374.

[9] H.B. Biller, *Paternal Deprivation.*

[10] W.A. Barry, "Marriage Research and Conflict: An Integrative Review," pp. 41-55.

the boy is exposed to other disturbing husband-wife interactions, a distorted view of male-female relationships develops. The feminine is devalued and the boy restricts his development to an extreme and rigid male gender role.

By contrast, when the boy has both an involved and respected mother and an involved and respected father, he is then exposed to a wider degree of valued and adaptive characteristics. He feels pride in his basic sex-role orientation and comfortable enough in himself to be relatively flexible in his responses. Research indicates that a positive father-mother relationship results not only in healthy male role identification, but also leads to boys most able to combine a positive masculinity with generally androgynous patterns of social interaction.[11] Boys capable of androgyny had fathers who were not only masculine, but participated in the normally "feminine" role of child care, displayed to their sons the normally "feminine" qualities of emotion and expressiveness, and were supportive and valuing of their wives and of the mother-child relationship.

In essence, the road to the nontraditional androgynous male who can accept traditionally feminine qualities is not through a diminishment in his masculinity, but through a secure self-confidence in that role which permits him also to feel comfortable with qualities traditionally associated with the feminine.

Parenthetically, girls who displayed a positive androgyny in their sex-role behavior seemed to be influenced by the behavior of both parents. Their fathers were warm, had positive views toward females and consistently encouraged independence and achievement; their mothers were likely to be working and also encouraged independence.[12] Parental encouragement of these qualities and a lack of rigid restriction does seem especially important if young girls are to develop competence in intellectual and physical endeavors.

Psychological research indicates that a high level of gender role typing is not desirable. For example, high femininity in females has

---

[11] E.M. Hetherington, M. Cox and R. Cox, "Family Interaction and the Social, Emotional and Cognitive Development of Children Following Divorce."

[12] H.B. Biller, *Paternal Deprivation;* H.B. Biller and D.L. Meredith, *Father Power.*

consistently been correlated with high anxiety, low self-esteem, and low social acceptance; and, although high masculinity in males has been correlated during adolescence with better psychological adjustment, it has been correlated during adulthood with high anxiety, high neuroticism and low self-acceptance.[13] Males and females who are more gender typed have been found to have lower overall intelligence, lower spatial ability and lower creativity.[14]

My own clinical experience corroborates this psychological research and indicates that many conflicts men have around the issue of masculine identity result from inappropriate gender identification. I shall discuss four such situations:

1. A defensive masculine identification due to an absent father and an intrusive mother.

2. A developmental overidentification with the masculine role that leads to loss of individuality and lack of generational conflict.

3. A competitive father who castrates his son's masculinity.

4. A masculine overidentification combined with a devaluation of the feminine.

Separation from the Mother

A common archetypal motif is that of the hero's struggle for separation from the Great Mother. This theme has been psychologically interpreted by Jung as a paradigm of the ego's differentiation from the unconscious.[15] Concretely, it manifests in efforts to separate one's individuality from various identifications.

The earliest identification is with the primary caretaker, usually the mother. As noted above in chapter four, in the discussion on separation anxiety, separating from the mother creates anxiety due to the child's awareness of its helpless state. The father plays a vital role in

---

[13] M.D. Gall, "The Relationship Between Masculinity-Femininity and Manifest Anxiety," pp. 294-295; T.C. Hartford, C.H. Willis and H.L. Deabler, "Personality Correlates of Masculinity-Femininity," pp. 881-884; P.H. Mussen, "Some Antecedents and Consequents of Masculine Sex-Typing in Adolescent Boys," p. 506; P.H. Mussen, "Long-Term Consequents of Masculinity of Interests in Adolescence," pp. 435-440.

[14] E.E. Maccoby, "Sex Differences in Intellectual Functioning."

[15] *Symbols of Transformation*, CW 5, pars. 539-540, 548.

this process. If he is receptive and supportive as the child moves away from the mother, the child will want to identify with him as an alternative. The father's role is to draw the child into the real world of things and people. He helps the child differentiate from the mother by representing the wider world that the child is entering.

In terms of gender identity, the father functions as the primary representative of the outer world, defining acceptable gender roles for daughters as well as sons. The father's failure to fulfill this role has different significance for the boy and the girl. If a young girl remains identified with her mother she suffers a loss of individuality in terms of her feminine development. She has a female identity, but it is a replication of her mother's. A boy, on the other hand, has to switch his primary identification from that of a female to that of a male, otherwise he loses his gender identity.

The importance of the father in helping a boy separate from his earliest identification with the mother and give him a male identity is seen in the puberty initiation rituals of so-called primitive societies.[16] Common to these rituals is the separation of the young adolescent from his mother, who ritually mourns the son as if he were dead. The boy is isolated among the males, often for months or years, where he undergoes a period of instruction characterized by various ordeals. During this period the he is taught his adult male role. When he returns to the tribe the boy is now considered a man and usually lives in the men's house.

These initiation rituals emphasize the importance for boys of breaking the connection with mother in learning to be men. A man gets his masculine identification in the company of other men, not from relationships with women. When a mother is intrusive and controlling and the father, due to absence, indifference or weakness, does not fulfill his initiatory function of helping his son separate, the boy's masculine development is disturbed. Not only does he not develop a secure masculine gender role, but the inner image of the feminine, the anima, fails to adequately differentiate from the image of the mother. The male does not grow up free to experience women as something other than the dominating femininity of the mother.

---

16 M. Eliade, *Rites and Symbols of Initiation.*

A common problem that develops in such circumstances is an unconscious fear of being feminine, overcompensated by a defensive masculine role, as if by the sheer extremeness of the masculine role the boy tries to overwhelm the feared feminine control. Proving that they are not effeminate is a major preoccupation of such paternally deprived males. They compulsively reject anything they perceive as related to femininity. Their fear of a female identification contributes to their need to control anything feminine, inside or outside themselves. Such defensively masculine men frequently engage in a Don Juan pattern of behavior, defining and exhibiting their masculinity by their relationships with women, for instance by how many different women they can have sex with.

Common to these men is what the psychoanalyst Ethel Person calls the fantasy of the "omni-available woman."[17] This fantasy is characterized by a woman who is always available sexually, forever lubricated, forever ready, forever desiring. It suggests an overabundance of women whose primary interest and sole function is sexual, ensuring that the man will never be humiliated. They are completely under the man's control, always willing and never rejecting. The women are automatically satisfied and require no special stimulus. Since these women are easy to please and experience great pleasure they assuage a man's self-doubt.

A man I will call Robert came to therapy because of a need to dominate women. In addition to compulsive masturbatory fantasies of the omni-available woman, Robert was involved in sado-masochistic sex. Any self-assertion by a woman threatened his male self-image and he responded with rage and control. His primary intent, however, was not to hurt the woman, only to have her recognize his power and masculinity.

Robert's father had left the family to fight in World War Two shortly after Robert was born. His mother and father had decided to marry and have a child after the father realized he was to be inducted. The child was to "remind" the wife of her husband while he was gone. The mother, who had hoped for a quiet daughter to keep her company, insisted on calling her son Roberta.

---

[17] "The Omni-Available Woman and Lesbian Sex: Two Fantasy Themes and Their Relationship to the Male Developmental Experience."

Robert's father returned home safely from the war when Robert was four years old. However, he was a passive man easily dominated by his wife and spent as little time at home as possible. The marriage did not work and by the time Robert was eight the parents divorced. Robert's mother solaced her feelings of abandonment and loneliness through her son. She continually discouraged signs of separation and masculine development in Robert, not allowing him to play ball or running games with the neighborhood boys. Instead she would insist that he play quietly in the house or help her with the cooking.

During the fifth grade Robert missed so much school due to "sickness" that the school administration asked that he and his mother meet with the school psychologist. It became clear that Robert's absences from school began when he developed some minor ailment and his mother treated it with exaggerated importance. Robert was kept at home, ostensibly to convalesce, but was gradually presented with a picture of himself as being unfit for the rough world of school and, therefore, in constant need of his mother's care. Unkind teachers, bullying boys and chronic ill health were inculpated as the villains of the piece.

When Robert reached adolescence he rebelled against his mother's attempts at domination. Rather than the sensitive, introverted person she had encouraged him to be, he overcompensated, forcing himself to be extroverted and athletic. To be masculine became an obsession with Robert. He broke bones and acquired scars in sports at which he was never proficient. As an adult he impaired his health on daring exploratory trips into the jungles of Brazil; he took up parachuting and learned to sky-dive. He made a career of conquering and abandoning women. Any sign of emotion was quickly squelched for fear of losing his precarious masculine identity. In defense against being dominated by his mother, he became a caricature of a man.

The initial phases of Robert's therapy were characterized by him parading his sexual conquests for my admiration. These episodes were especially extreme when he felt insecure in the face of feminine assertion or if he had experienced "feminine" feelings of affection or intimacy. In his fantasy, I admired and valued his dominating behavior, respected his macho masculinity and was somewhat envious of his conquests and control over women.

During this period, I had various countertransference reactions to Robert. I felt the desire to educate him about male-female relationships, to instruct him on the proper way to treat women. Once I actually acted this out and suggested he treat a particular woman more as an equal. My remark was met with a tirade about weak men castrated by women. At other times, I identified with his projected father and felt unmasculine, and once even wondered if I should have an affair to prove my masculinity.

During his second year of therapy, while sitting in the waiting room, a female analyst from an adjacent office replaced a picture on the waiting room wall with a new one. Robert stormed into his session muttering about "dominating bitches who feel they have the right to control everybody." "Everybody," in this instance, turned out to be me, the passive wimp. "Why do you let the bitch next door control you?" he demanded. "What right did she have to replace your picture with hers, and not even ask permission? Her personality is taking over and you are too weak to even care. I bet you're dominated by your wife at home."

After this tirade, I suggested that the waiting room was like his young personality, which had been intruded on and dominated by his mother, and he was angry because he felt I was like his father, incapable of asserting myself and rescuing his masculinity from his mother. The session ended in silence.

During the next week Robert had three dreams which helped him realize what he feared and struggled against.

There is a dog on a tight leash led by a lady. I feel that the dog is myself. I'm furious at being tied to my mother. I can't tell whether the dog is male or female.

I'm going to a Caribbean Island for a vacation. A fat, butch, dyke-type woman in authority won't let me on the airplane even though I'm in the front of the line and there are seats. I'm full of rage but feel weak and helpless to do anything about it. I'm wearing a dress.

Inside a fence is a monster animal. It is me. Some women outside the fence are making me fight with another beast. It was for their amusement. I kept running around saying: "Do I have to? Please don't make me do it!" I'd run back and fight and then run back and say: "Please no more." Then one of the women said: "Here's your reward. You can play with your little tin can." So I played with it like a little puppy and then they made me go back and fight again. She was making me do it to entertain them.

In his analysis of these dreams it became clear to Robert that his fantasy of the "omni-available woman," as well as his sado-masochistic sexual domination, were forms of magical repair of his damaged masculinity and fear of femininity. While he acted out wishful fantasies about size, hardness, endurance, skill and willing females, his fears were typical of the brittle masculinity of the man afraid of feminine control: impotence, lack of skill, rejection and homosexual dread. He attempted to assuage his masculine self-doubt through the collective male fantasy of machismo, in which control over the feared woman is sought through sexual mastery.

I pointed out to Robert that what was missing in the dreams was a strong masculine presence. The dreams consisted solely of Robert and powerful women. There was no male figure to nurture, protect and guide him.

My observation helped Robert begin to realize that rather than demeaning his father, he really wanted to idealize him. Similarly, rather than putting me down, Robert wanted me to be the strong man who would initiate him into manhood and rescue him from his fear of being the girl his mother always wanted. The insight that what he really wanted was a closer relationship with me aroused a new level of anxiety. The desire for intimacy and affection with another man implied that he was homosexual, and that his mother had actually succeeded in turning him into a woman. In addition, he imagined that I was repulsed by his need for intimacy and would humiliate him. During this period Robert experienced the depths of the masculine insecurity that underlay his dominating masculine role.

One night Robert dreamed:

I am playing ball with a man. The game is competitive but not aggressive. He is better at the game than I. I hope the other man will be my friend. I want his company and help. Perhaps he'll teach me.

After this dream, new fantasies began to emerge of him and me doing active things together. Robert began to imagine us doing carpentry or playing golf, activities at which, in his imagination, I was proficient and aided his development.

When Robert's feelings of intimacy first began to emerge, my countertransference matched his feared expectation. I was upset with myself over my hostile feelings and my thoughts of how weak and needy he was. It was only after I could disidentify from his projection of the macho masculine image and connect to my own feelings of being a nurturing father, that I could accept and lovingly relate to his tentative reaching for a masculine guide.

Overidentification with Traditional Masculine Values

I have mentioned that in mythology the hero's fight with the Great Mother is symbolic of the individual's struggle to break free of various identifications, the first of which is with the personal mother. For the development of individuality, however, a person needs not only to separate from the mother; a heroic fight with the father must also take place.

In mythology, the father is often symbolic of the old order and the young hero is representative of the new. Fathers represent and reinforce the religious, ethical, political and social values of the collective. The outer father and the inner father image are conditioned by the character of the culture transmitting these values. As noted earlier, research shows that fathers exert a greater effect than mothers on the formation of gender roles for both sons and daughters. Mothers tend to treat their children the same, without regard to whether the child is male or female. Fathers, on the other hand, in their concern for society's standards, tend to reinforce the instrumental dimension in boys and the expressive dimension in girls.

The danger is that the father may fix consciousness in the wrong direction by upholding the old system of values. Fathers impress the values of their generation on the young. Those who identify with these values are included among the adults. While this breaks the unconscious identification with the mother, it is replaced by an unconscious identification with traditional masculine values. There results a stable sameness between culture, parent and child that is devoid of generational conflict. People who are completely identified with convention and collective norms via identification with the father are castrated. They cannot develop into individuals. They merely live out what has always been. I'll give two examples of patriarchal castration in terms of male psychology.

In the Old Testament Book of Genesis the story is told of Abraham and Isaac. Abraham was an old man, a hundred, when his wife Sarah became pregnant with Isaac. Abraham loved this child of his old age. To test Abraham's faith, God ordered him to sacrifice Isaac. Abraham went to the mountain God had directed him to, built an altar, piled it high with firewood and tied Isaac to the top. As he reached for the knife to plunge into his son, God intervened and told Abraham to stop, he had proven his fear of God. Then a ram appeared, caught in a bush, and Abraham sacrificed the ram in place of his son. As a result of this proof of his obedience to God, Abraham was promised that his descendants would be a mighty people.

This story is usually told to provide an example of Abraham's faith in God. I like to think of it from the point of view of Isaac, as an example of how a son's individuality is castrated by a developmental overidentification with his father. Isaac shows complete and utter reliance on his father. After all, God did not order Isaac to kill himself. He ordered Abraham to sacrifice Isaac. Thus Isaac was subject to his father's relationship to God and his father's spiritual values, not his own.

Isaac's position is in many ways quite natural. It is normal for a son to want to be like his father; he feels proud when he can be accepted by other adult males as a man just like his father. The positive benefits of such developmental identification are the transmission of collective cultural values, acceptance by society, a secure identity and inclusion among the adults. An inability to successfully identify brings feelings of inferiority, shame and betrayal.

In Western societies, we have few meaningful rituals to help in the transition to an adult masculine identity. However, initiation is an archetypal dynamic that causes a person to unconsciously seek initiation wherever possible so transitions can properly occur.

A colleague told me that one of the things that made him proud as an adolescent was working with his father, a peasant immigrant from Russia, on his furniture moving truck. They worked sixteen hours a day, six days a week. No matter how exhausted they were, no matter how much their bodies hurt, neither ever complained. He remembered how great it felt as a boy to be a man like his father. Only years later did he realize that he had been initiated into the masculinity of a Russian peasant. He remained unconsciously identified with that collective peasant identity of physical toil until his early thirties when he went to live on a mountain and spent untold hours cutting and chopping firewood. He realized then, with a great sense of betraying his father, that he hated being like that. He really was not meant to be a beast of burden. He valued consciousness and psychological development, not the activity-based masculinity of his father.

I once knew a man named Frank who was a tremendous athlete. He played baseball so superbly that he was offered a contract to play in the farm system of the New York Mets. Frank idealized his father who was a carpenter. He asked his father whether or not to take the offer. His father said there was an opening in the carpenter's union, a rare event, and that he could get his son the slot. He advised his son to take the secure union job, rather than risk the uncertainty of a baseball career.

Frank followed his father's suggestion. Years later I asked Frank, by then thirty years old, married with children and playing ball for barroom teams, how he now felt about the decision he made. Frank said his decision was based on love for his father; his father was his idol and Frank wanted to be just like him. Besides, to do otherwise would have been a betrayal, a statement that his father's way was not good enough. Continuing his father's life had been Frank's way of avoiding the guilt of betrayal. However, Frank said he was no longer sure he had made the right decision.

Another form of patriarchal castration, a reaction to the Isaac complex, is the permanent revolutionary. While this type of man appears to be a hero who is always slaying the dragon of authority and tradition, he is really a false hero. He rebels against authority simply because authority is associated with the father, not because he has come to an individual position. A man of this kind can never assume power himself, never be a father. He is tied to the old values by always having to rebel against them. He cannot come to a true position of his own.

Along with betrayal and guilt, fear of deviance, with its attendant feelings of inadequacy and shame, prevents men from defining their masculine identity in a way that differs from that of the father and the collective.

Fear of deviance is a fear of engaging in behavior that contradicts culturally learned norms and thereby threatens sex-role identity. Fear of deviance is based on realistic experiences of negative consequences. The actual consequences of deviance can account for the fear of it and result in an urge toward conformity. Fear of deviance causes men to avoid certain goals—emotional and psychological development, for example—which they consider unmasculine.

An analysand I will call Stan refused to show any feelings except anger toward his family or friends. His wife was threatening to leave the marriage because of what she called his emotional shallowness. Coming to therapy was a last, shameful and desperate attempt on Stan's part to change. However, he could no more show or discuss his feelings with me than with others.

During the third month of therapy Stan had an anxiety attack in the waiting room before his session. He thought of walking out and leaving a note saying he would never return. Instead, he waited and started the session in his usual hostile manner, criticizing my attire and professional competence. Finally, as he began to discuss the frightening experience he had had in the waiting room, he realized that he had begun to trust and like me over the last few months. This aroused the fear of needing me, feeling dependent and showing feelings.

"Why should that frighten you?" I asked.

Stan got red in the face and his voice started to tremble. "I might cry," he said, "and you would make fun of me."

Stan then told of painful experiences in his childhood when his father and older brother teased him unmercifully for crying, calling him "sissy" and "fairy." Real men, they said, controlled themselves and did not act weak. Stan naturally identified with their viewpoint and developed a hatred of his own sensitive, emotional nature. Any behavior that was not stereotypically masculine became feminine. Rather than study art, he chose his father's "more masculine" craft of plumbing.

As he grew older Stan's fears of not being masculine developed into a fear of homosexuality. In his therapy, he was terrified of two things. The first was that if he showed his feelings I would consider him gay and humiliate and reject him. The second, and even more frightening fear, was that I was really homosexual and was trying to seduce him. With great shame, he told me that he had often wondered about my sexuality. I seemed to be a warm, sensitive person; I encouraged him to express his feelings and did not respond to his viselike handshake by increasing the pressure of my own. These were behaviors that, if he did them himself, would cause him to feel nonmasculine.

Some men who recognize the limitations of the narrow masculine role in which they have been raised worry that if they give it up they will be rejected by women. While this is often due to the projection of their own fears, in many instances it is an accurate perception of conflicts women have about men. Despite protestations to the contrary, many women are conflicted about their desire to relate to nontraditional men. On the one hand, they desire a man who is open, sensitive, related and egalitarian. On the other hand, due to their own father identifications, they want a man who embodies the traditional masculine values of strength, independence and invulnerability.

One woman I worked with in psychotherapy provides an example of how such a conflict can affect both men and women.

My patient had married a man who, like her traditional father, was cold and withdrawn and did not believe in displaying weakness. She complained endlessly about her husband's unwillingness to share his anxieties and conflicts. As a result of his own therapy, the man slowly began to change. He recognized his insecurity and vulnerability and began to speak to his wife about these parts of himself. Was she happy? Yes, on the surface. But she had a way of making hurtful comments every time he revealed himself. When he complained to her about this she declared him to be oversensitive and defensive, further alienating him and forcing him back into his cold, withdrawn position.

Meanwhile, my analysand's dreams revealed that she was conflicted about her husband's change. His insecurity aroused dependency conflicts which lay hidden behind the traditional roles she and her husband lived. If her husband was weak then she would have to assume more responsibility and let him lean on her.

On one level , this woman wanted to be stronger and more independent; on another, she took comfort in her traditional feminine position of passivity and having a "strong" man around to take care of her. Also, she unconsciously identified with her father. While she had adopted an egalitarian rhetoric, she really believed that masculinity, which she defined in terms of her father's silent, strong and controlling behavior, was superior. Femininity was considered weak and submissive. When her husband revealed his fears, in her mind he became a weak, inferior woman. She, in turn, became the superior, aggressive male and derived great unconscious satisfaction from her subtle sadistic comments.

In mythology, real heroes fight the father to attain their own destiny and true nature, not as a mere reaction. They follow an inner voice that tells them of a new way to live. It is because they listen to this inner voice and want the world to change that they become breakers of the old law and enemies of the ruling system. Thus they come into conflict with the "fathers" and their spokesman, the personal father. The inner voice they listen to is their own nature. Their consciousness is expanded by a new idea, a new conception of how things can be, and they, as heroes, have the courage to follow this apprehension. As soon as they listen to themselves, as soon as they honor their individuality, they are psychologically in conflict with the father world.

This is a struggle we all must go through in our personal development. A man must separate his conscious personality from that of his father's way of being male, and a woman must separate her sense of the masculine from unconscious identification with father. To not separate means to live a limited life.

Competition with the Father

There is a form of castration which is the inadvertent result of a too loving developmental identification between father and son. The father's intent is not to harm his son; his desire is simply to have his son be a man like himself, a desire the son shares out of love and admiration for his father.

The Kronus myth, on the other hand, describes castration due to a competitive father-son relationship. In this story, Uranus, jealous of his sons, thrust them deep beneath the earth. Gaia, wife of Uranus, angry at her husband's behavior, produced a sickle of steel which one of her sons, Kronus, used to castrate his father. Kronus, now in charge, also feared his children and swallowed each at birth. Rhea, sister of Kronus and mother of his children, deceived Kronus by substituting a rock for her youngest child Zeus who, when he grew to maturity, overthrew his father.

A significant characteristic of the male gender role is to be successful in the outer world. But this requires the ability to be competitive and the controlled utilization of assertion and aggression, qualities also associated with the masculine role. Anything that interferes with the development of these qualities, in men or women, will also impede their chances for worldly success.

A significant failure in the adaptation of men who fear success is inhibition of competitiveness and aggression. The developmental origin of such inhibitions is often early rivalries between the child and its father or siblings. If the father is competitive with his children, the child's normal rivalry is heightened. Some fathers humiliate their sons when they compete. Others arouse guilt or threaten withdrawal. Where there is severe intimidation, the equation between aggression and violence is reinforced. The child begins to withhold aggression out of fear of violent retaliation. The misconception that aggression must be violent is extended to assertion of all kinds. As an adult with ambitions intact, but aggression inhibited, the person lacks the capacity to take effective action. Competition is associated with the original rivalries of childhood. The attitudes toward the father become transferred to other men. Open recognition of interest in success for these persons carries with it the potential risk of retaliation by the parental competitor.

For men, the major forms of unconscious fantasized retaliation are castration and homosexual submission. Since, in our society, masculinity is associated with strength and superiority, it is not surprising that people who suffer from conflicts over aggression and competition often associate success and decisiveness with phallic potency, which in turn is associated concretely with the penis. For them, being successful means having a large, "adult" penis. Having an adult penis, however, arouses unconscious competition with the father. The resultant castration anxiety is defended against by self-castration. They experience and present themselves as not having an adult penis. Sometimes this manifests as a fantasy that their penis is too small to satisfy a woman; at other times, they may be beset with homosexual fantasies. Both fantasies lead to anxiety symptoms, which often become accentuated after a successful experience.

An analysand who worked as a therapist had the above symptoms. He was afraid to progress in his own therapy or show his interest in professional subjects. He fantasized that I would experience his ambition to become an expert therapist as competition for masculine supremacy and that I would try to hurt him. This caused him to hide his professional and psychological growth. Instead, he revealed to me only his conflicts and weaknesses.

This man also fantasized that I was having affairs with my patients. Ultimately, he began an affair with the patient of another analyst. He suffered great anxiety telling me about this and fantasized that I was angry. His associations indicated that he unconsciously considered his affair a victory over me and associated his success with having an adult penis. This revealed his competitiveness with me. He wanted to become an expert in order to be a better analyst than I was. His fantasy was that then all my patients would come to him, especially the women. He further imagined that he and I would display our penises and the women would consider his larger and more attractive. In the fantasy, I became enraged and threatened him with a meat cleaver. He felt defenseless. Having an adult penis placed him in competition with me, the analyst/father, and constellated castration fear. He defended against this by presenting himself in a castrated manner, hiding his potency.

Consistent interpretation of this man's fear of success in terms of his fear of competing with his father was followed by a dream:

> I find my stolen shoes in a homosexual's shoe store. After I retrieved my shoes I was attacked by a bully with yellow hair who hit me on the buttocks with a tool.

He associated his shoes to his ability to maintain a phallic stand-point, and the yellow hair to a lion and then to his father who is a Leo. He experienced the dream as confirming his fear of being potently masculine. During the following weeks he began to experience irrational anger toward male figures on the street. This subsequently turned into directed, assertive feelings toward the abusive director of the mental health clinic where he worked. In time, he became able to experience his own ambitions separate from his competitive feelings toward others and free of unreasonable anxiety.

Awareness of competitiveness and self-assertion not only arouses fear of retaliation, but, since it is symbolically equated with the fantasized murder of one's parent, it also arouses guilt. The consequent need to inhibit assertion can in turn lead to phobic behavior. If success is achieved, the need to undo the guilt, through penance of some kind, can result in self-punishment or masochistic adaptations.

The unconscious need for punishment may not be connected to actual misdeeds, but simply to fantasies or wishes that are deemed immoral. We see this in people who inflict unnecessary injury on themselves, fail in their careers when they are about to succeed or cannot let themselves enjoy anything. One man's father died when he was four. He fantasized that his sexual desire for his mother and aggressive thoughts about the father had sickened and killed the father. He felt he had won his mother but was guilty of patricide. Thus he experienced terrible guilt whenever he successfully asserted himself. Feeling that he did not deserve to live for his heinous crime, he supposed that his life should be one of atonement through suffering.

Analysts are vulnerable to a particular countertransference reaction toward analysands working through conflicts centered around competition and self-assertion. The analyst might identify with the castrating aggression of the projected father-image and force interpretations. In such a case, the analysand could be afraid to assert his potency against what he experiences as the father/analyst's demands for submission. Instead, he resists the analyst and simultaneously competes with him by failing. If the analyst remains unaware of the dynamics involved, frustration over the lack of progress in the analysis can result in even more forceful interpretations.

A man in therapy with me had been continually humiliated and castrated by the intellect of his professor father. For instance, the father would insist on editing his son's school reports and then take credit for his excellent grades. As a result of identifying with the patient, I began to feel impotent. I tried to regain my supremacy by dominating, insisting on the correctness of my interpretations (which in fact, I later realized, were abstract and theoretical). The patient responded to my aggressive competition the same way he had with his father; he identified with me as the aggressor and proceeded to satisfy my need for power by attributing his successes to me rather than to himself. He escaped castration fear by experiencing success not as his own but as due to my imagined attributes.

Since assertion in our culture is associated with the male gender role, women have a complicated relationship to achievement that often centers around the symbol of masculinity, the penis and concerns about femininity.

In patriarchal families, where favoritism is displayed toward a male child, the father is very dominant or the mother and femininity are devalued, a young girl naturally develops the wish to be male. This wish tends to center on the penis itself, not because she actually desires to have the physical organ, but because it is the significantly different feature which to her mind would explain the different way in which she is regarded. It is the symbolic equivalent of the penis—especially strength, aggression, domination, power and success—that is valued, due to the erroneous relationship established between value and masculinity. Since father or brother have the penis that is symbolically desired, it can only be obtained via their castration. In such circumstances, a woman can develop a fear of retaliation from men whenever she tries to be successful.

A female analysand was the third child in a patriarchal family. There were two older brothers. Her fear of success manifested in her working as a file clerk after quitting college in her third year despite being an above average student. Neither brother went to college and both worked as construction laborers like the father. The analysand had always felt unloved and unvalued. She had the feeling she was defective in some way and if she could only find out what she was missing she'd be able to make it right.

As a child she tried to urinate standing up and would get angry if her mother tried to make her sit down. She had been constipated, was a tomboy who beat up all the boys in the neighborhood but never fought with the girls. One day one of the boys took out his penis and urinated on her. This devastated her and she became deeply depressed. Her memory of these childhood experiences led to the following associations.

Standing up and urinating was the way boys did it. Her constipated feces had the shape of a penis; to hold a turd was a way of having a penis and being a boy. To beat up the boys was to symbolically become a boy because aggression and dominance were associated with phallic power. She did not beat up the girls because boys did not fight with girls. She was depressed by the boy who urinated on her because she could not take out her own penis and return his aggression. In addition, and most painful of all, was the feeling that if she had been a boy her parents would have loved and valued her like her brothers.

During the period of our discussions, she dreamed:

I see a stretch limousine and admire how long and powerful it is. I feel envious of the successful man who owns it. Then I realize it belongs to me and feel nervous. It is too valuable. Somebody might try to steal it, especially if it is left on the street. Besides, it's too big. I don't think I could drive it properly. Behind the limo is a little Volkswagon Beetle. That's more like it. It would be much safer to own that car. Easier to drive and nobody else would want it.

This dream confirmed that the symbolic equation she had unconsciously developed around the issue of success was: "If I am successful, then I must be a man and have a penis. If I have a penis I must have obtained it by stealing it from one of my brothers who will seek retaliation. I will be safer if I am smaller and less noticeable."

In addition, she realized that because of the mistaken association between assertion, goal achievement and masculinity, being successful aroused shame and inferiority over not being as feminine as her mother. She unconsciously knew that being successful as something other than a housewife and mother was not what her father expected of her. Whenever this quite talented woman approached the successful achievement of her goals, these fantasies were activated. They generated fear, a sense of inadequacy and shame.

Homoerotic Anxiety

In the previous section I discussed the castrating effect on a woman of being raised in an environment which overvalues traditional masculine qualities, undervalues feminine qualities and sharply differentiates these into gender roles. Here I will describe the possible effect of such an environment on a man.

Over the years I have encountered in my clinical work a significant number of men who suffer from what I call homoerotic anxiety. They are not homosexual. Homosexuals are considered to be men who have a predominant romantic and sexual relationship with other men. Even where they live a heterosexual life, they are aware that their primary attraction is to other men. By contrast, men who experience homoerotic anxiety enjoy sexual relationships with women, have never, or rarely, had sex with men and yet experience anxiety about the possibility of being homosexual.

The traditional Jungian position on male homosexuality is that the normal archetypal relationship in the family is reversed due to a predominant influence of the feminine. If this leads to a pathological dependency on the feminine, there develops an identification of the ego with the anima. Longing for masculine guidance, the young male overcompensates by associating only with men, as if to reinforce the male principle in the face of the original overweighting of the female. Essentially, then, homosexuality is an attempt to overcome, via compensation, a matriarchal psychology where the Great Mother is unconsciously in the ascendant. This view can be amplified by how exclusively male societies originate under matriarchal conditions in an attempt to overcome the supremacy of the matriarchate.

While explaining some forms of homosexuality, the pattern of a weak unmasculine father combined with an overly intense and exclusive mother-son relationship is not the case in homoerotic anxiety. Clinical material gathered from the analysis of a number of male patients indicates that it results from the one-sided identification with a limited masculine viewpoint and consequent rejection of the feminine. These men were all raised in an environment where the women were essentially weak, dependent, nurturing, servants to dominating, physically powerful, tough men who lacked feeling, creativity and spontaneity. The patients strongly identified with this limited image of the masculine. There was no question of inner feminine or contrasexuality. Rather than the normal archetypal family relationship being reversed, as it may be in the development of homosexuals, it was exaggerated.

Symptomatically, homoerotic anxiety intruded into the conscious lives of these individuals in an obsessive and compulsive manner. Typically, they found themselves compelled to look at the genital area of other men or they wondered how big their penis was compared to others. For instance, one patient refused to join a health club for fear that he would not be able to avoid staring at other men's penises in the locker room.

All these men feared affection for other men as a sign of homosexuality and defended against their fears by paranoid thoughts of other men coming on to them. Quite naturally, this affects the transference relationship with male analysts.

A twenty-five-year-old patient I will call Sam had an irrational fear of being attacked by strangers on the street. During one session, he reacted with hostility to what I considered a series of helpful and correct interventions. When I pointed out his anger Sam said he experienced my interpretations as hostilely motivated and refused to be affected by them. Subsequently, he dreamed of a black man stabbing him in the back. I suggested that he was afraid of being penetrated from the rear in an aggressive manner and that he experienced my interventions not as a helpful act but as a form of homosexual rape.

Reluctantly, Sam admitted that he had felt warm, grateful feelings for me after my previous interpretations. But he had also been upset by the fact that I leaned forward as I made my comments. Both his feelings and my physical movement had been assimilated by his homoerotic complex. Sam understood his warm feelings as a homosexual reaction. My leaning forward was distorted into an invitation to closer physical intimacy. These erotic feelings and fantasies were then defended by anger.

Sam's paranoid defenses kept him always on guard against my discovering his secrets. During one session he embarrassedly described a fantasy he had had the previous evening when he heard the elevator door in the building of his residence open onto his floor.

Sam had imagined I was sneaking down the hallway in order to listen at his door and discover him doing something illegal. He, in turn, would quietly approach and open the door in order to catch me spying. When I commented that the theme of the fantasy was his being caught at some illicit activity, he immediately associated to the discovery of homoerotic feelings.

Angry thoughts about women also aroused anxiety in these men that they were homosexual. They understood their devaluation of women as a general hatred of them, which they assumed indicated that they really wanted to be with a man. Sam, for instance, treated his previous female analyst with the disdain reserved for the depreciated women in his personal background. According to Sam, she became enraged by his demeaning behavior and attacked his masculinity, telling him that his behavior indicated he was really defending against homosexual urges. Her retaliatory aggression terrified Sam and further aroused his homoerotic anxiety, not only because of her angry declaration about his feared homosexuality, but because his fear of her indicated to Sam that he was not as powerful with women as his dominant father and so must be homosexual.

I will try to explain the relationship I have noticed between a rigid male gender role, devalued femininity and homoerotic anxiety.

Jung assumed that a primary motivation in the psyche is the instinctive drive for wholeness, the union of opposites. One manifestation of this is the drive to unite masculine and feminine elements in the personality.[18] For a man, Jung believed that the symbolic goal of union can only be concretely achieved if those attributes that exist as unconscious potential in the anima are integrated by the ego. But how is this possible when what is associated with the feminine has been devalued and rejected by a rigid and one-sided view of the masculine?

So far I have discussed the anima as a symbol of undeveloped potential in a man, as a repository for aspects of the total personality that a man is not allowed to recognize or develop due to the limitations of gender identity. However, as an archetype the anima is more than just a structure housing undeveloped contents, it is also a dy-

---

18 See "The Psychology of the Transference," *The Practice of Psychotherapy*, CW 16, esp. pars. 410-449 and figure 2, p. 213.

namism that is teleologically oriented, that is, the anima has an instinctive goal. Jung goes so far as to suggest recognizing the anima as an autonomous personality with a will of her own.[19]

If we assume that the anima's goal is to fulfill the psyche's drive toward wholeness, then we would expect that those undeveloped qualities associated with the anima would be driven toward union with the masculine ego-consciousness. Ideally, one would want this totality to be an intrapsychic phenomenon, an experience in which the masculine ego becomes aware of, embraces and develops the qualities symbolized by the anima.

However, if, because of the limitations imposed by a rigid gender identification, the anima's drive to achieve union is frustrated, it is possible that the anima might choose to satisfy its need for masculine connection elsewhere, perhaps by an attraction to another man.

Since constellated complexes and archetypes are accompanied by particular body and feeling sensations, the individual would experience a physical as well as a psychological attraction. While the psychologically naive individual would perceive only the phenomena of male/male interaction, the mediated psychological dynamic would be between inner feminine and outer masculine—a teleological drive for the totality symbolized as a union of masculine and feminine.

Let me illustrate with an example. In his third year of therapy, Sam had a dream in which a young, semideveloped female figure, whom Sam had earlier in the dream rejected, became interested in another man. Sam awoke filled with anxieties about homosexuality.

During his therapy session, Sam said the other man in the dream was a friend toward whom he had noticed erotic feelings. Sam said this man was effeminate, which turned out to mean he was vulnerable, open with his feelings and had a respectful relationship with his girlfriend. Sam then engaged the female dream figure in an active imagination. Rather than rejecting her as he had in the dream, he accepted her into a relationship and they had a dialogue. In brief, she told Sam that they both needed to grow and could only do so in a relationship. If Sam refused to relate to her then she would find another man to take his place, but she had to develop.

---

[19] "The Relations Between the Ego and the Unconscious," *Two Essays on Analytical Psychology,* CW 7, pars. 296-340.

As Sam sat quietly reflecting on this he realized that the attraction toward his friend was not his, but hers. Sam merely identified with the affect that took place in the common physical and psychological home that he and the anima shared.

Sam then had a kind of fantasy vision during which he experienced a swirling mass of energy that he knew was the essence of femininity. This energy filled him with such an empty cavernous ache that he despaired of ever filling it. This was a part of his essential being. Another swirl of energy then flowed directly into the first, filling it completely and perfectly. Sam knew that was the essence of masculinity. Then came the intuitive realization that the driving force behind his homoerotic fears was the need for the feminine to be filled and completed by the masculine, a need that was being ignored by a one-sided identification with a limited and rigid masculine viewpoint that depreciated the feminine.

This numinous experience was a projection of what Jung called the divine syzygy, the tendency for masculine and feminine images to occur together.[20] It had a healing effect and led to Sam's successful effort to change his attitude toward the feminine, both in his interpersonal relationships and with his inner woman. Step by step, with the relaxing of his rigid gender identity and the differentiation and integration of the anima, Sam experienced a diminution of his homoerotic anxiety.

---

20 "The Syzygy: Anima and Animus," *Aion*, CW 9ii.

7
Depression

Depression can be either normal or pathological. Normal depression is a natural reaction of the personality; it is appropriate in certain circumstances and is transitory. Like anxiety, in certain circumstances depression can become a disorder with specific mechanisms and dynamics. There is then a predisposition to depression, and this is one of the main discriminants between normal depression and the disordered variety. The same event may precipitate either. In normal depression the mood passes. In pathological depression it sets off the predisposition.

For the purpose of discussion, pathological depression will be differentiated into simple and melancholic.

When people suffer from a simple depression they do not want the depressed mood, feel it inappropriate to their life situation and try to fight it off. The mood itself is characterized by feelings of weakness, lack of motivation, pessimism and loneliness. A negative view exists—of the world, themselves and the future.

Melancholic depression is characterized by a pervasive and overwhelming feeling of self-blame, hopelessness and self-depreciation. Such people suffer from disordered thought processes, psychomotor retardation and somatic dysfunctions. Their thoughts are gloomy and morbid. Ideas of guilt and sin lead to a desire for punishment. There is a real danger of suicide.

Part I. A Discussion of Jung's Views

Jung did not develop a systematic theory of depression but left ideas on the subject scattered throughout his writings. The aim of this section is to systematize and evaluate these ideas.

Jung explained depression in terms of concepts derived from his libido theory, which involves the distribution of energy in the psyche. Ego-consciousness normally has an appropriate supply of energy. When certain factors cause an excessive portion of this supply

119

to fall into the unconscious, ego-consciousness is depleted. Depression is the ego's experience of itself with a lack of energy. Jung wrote:

> The unconscious has simply gained an unassailable ascendency; it wields an attractive force that can invalidate all conscious contents— in other words, it can withdraw libido from the conscious world and thereby produce a "depression," an *abaissement du niveau mental.* . . . But as a result of this we must, according to the law of energy, expect an accumulation of value—i.e., libido—in the unconscious.[1]

Jung understood the dynamics of depression through the concepts of compensation and introversion. Compensation refers to the inherent self-regulation of the psyche. Only a limited number of contents can be held in consciousness at any one time and everything else is excluded as irrelevant. This makes the conscious orientation one-sided. The excluded contents form an unconscious counterposition, which, for an appropriate adaptation, is often necessary to balance or complement the conscious orientation.

Through the process of introversion, the contents that can compensate the one-sidedness of the ego are brought to consciousness. When libido introverts, it detaches itself from the object world and begins to activate the unconscious. This movement of energy depletes the ego and results in the experience of depression. When the unconscious contents are integrated, the ego is replenished by the energy symbolized by the contents as well as by the return of the introverting libido. Thus the depression is alleviated.

Jung saw a relationship between depression and transformation, and was primarily interested in applying his ideas about depression to the study of this relationship. For him the unconscious is creative, that is, it produces contents whose purpose is the development of the personality. The need to become aware of these issues may deprive the ego of energy and result in depression. In this case the depression is not a pathological reaction but a natural consequence of the inner need for transformation. In other words, being depressed is not necessarily a sign of neurosis.

---

[1] "The Relations Between the Ego and the Unconscious," *Two Essays on Analytical Psychology,* CW 7, par. 344.

In transformative depressions, libido is attracted by some psychic content that needs to become conscious in order to further the individuation process. This form of depression is purposive. The individual needs to reach a certain goal in development, and the unconscious element is necessary to achieve this; the depression becomes a means to that end. In order to recover the lost energy one must look into the unconscious and find what has attracted the energy. This attracting force will appear in the form of a fantasy or image. If the individual can bring up and integrate the images that attract and hold the libido, energy will again become available to ego-consciousness. Harding associates this pattern with a "creative depression."[2]

Myths of a hero's descent into the underworld in search of treasure are symbolic descriptions of entering the unconscious. The hero is a symbol of libido. When he enters the underworld we are presented with an image of depression as Jung conceives of it, a depletion of energy available to the ego to invest in the outer world. The hero's descent, according to Jung, is also a symbol of the process of introversion. Entering the underworld to fight a monster is psychologically equivalent to the ego coming to grips with an unconscious affect associated with a complex or archetype. Insofar as the hero is changed by this encounter, he "dies." Likewise the ego experiences death, preliminary to being born anew.

For example, the ego may hold a certain attitude about itself and the world, such as "everybody tries to take advantage of me because I am innocent and good." Through introversion the ego encounters a compensatory attitude, such as: "I take advantage of others." As a result, the paranoid view of the world is modified; the ego has been changed by the new attitude and its ramifications. With this restructuring the ego is reborn and the world is recreated. One feels differently about oneself and others, and relates differently.

The process of introversion is accompanied by depression for two reasons. The first is that the ego becomes depleted as its energy is drawn or directed toward the unconscious. The second is that all change has a component of permanent loss, usually symbolized by death and accompanied by depression. Just as this depression is a

---

[2] M. Esther Harding, "The Meaning and Value of Depression."

natural phenomenon, so is the other part of the transformation process, the emergence from depression with the experience of rebirth. The hero brings the treasure back to the surface. Psychologically, this means the ego has been remade by its encounter with the unconscious and this dispels the depression.

If one confuses the symbolic experience of death with physical death, there will be a resistance to the depression and its inherent goal of transformation.

For instance, an analysand going through an important experience of change that centered on the need to withdraw projections of his mother from his wife became hypochondriacal and paranoid. He began to wonder about carcinogens in the drinking water and fear the possibility of sudden death at the hands of muggers. When a cough refused to clear up, he developed the obsessive fantasy that he had terminal lung cancer. This symptom became so strong and the affect so real that even his wife, who was a physician, was convinced. For weeks he imagined he had no more than a few months to live. Only after associations to dream material connected his fear of dying to fear of psychological change did he realize its symbolic nature.

For most people, the depression that accompanies the loss of an old adaptation is a transitory event. One overcomes the fear of change and makes the required adaptation. Others suffer from depressive disorder and develop serious symptoms at the prospect of change or loss. For such people depression is not transient.

Jung attempted to explain depressive disorder with his ego-depletion theory, applying its concepts to simple depression, which he called psychogenic depression.

If the attitude of ego-consciousness becomes too one-sided and cannot be modified by normal compensation, a neurosis develops and the information that would compensate the conscious attitude is expressed through symptoms. Depressive disorder is the psyche's attempt to reorientate the personality toward an introverted experience. Pathological depression is thus an involuntary form of introversion.

In *Symbols of Transformation,* Jung gives an account of pathological depression as it relates to forced introversion:

The separation from youth has even taken away the golden glamour of Nature, and the future appears hopeless and empty. But what robs Nature of its glamour, and life of its joy, is the habit of looking back for something that used to be outside, instead of looking inside, into the depths of the depressive state. This looking back leads to regression and is the first step along that path. Regression is also an involuntary introversion in so far as the past is an object of memory and therefore a psychic content, an endopsychic factor. It is a relapse into the past caused by a depression in the present. Depression should therefore be regarded as an unconscious compensation whose content must be made conscious if it is to be fully effective. This can only be done by consciously regressing along with the depressive tendency and integrating the memories so activated into the conscious mind—which was what the depression was aiming at in the first place.[3]

In short, Jung considered depressive disorder to be a forced introversion serving the compensatory function. As a consequence of this the ego's energy is depleted. According to the principle of equivalence, the drawing off of libido from consciousness leads to an accumulation of energy in the unconscious.

Therapeutically, the disordered situation is treated by remedying the imbalance of energy in the psyche, not by looking for the cause of the depression in outer life. Since libido manifests as fantasy images, the imbalance can be rectified by bringing such images up from the unconscious and integrating them with the conscious mind. Jung wrote:

A causal explanation of these states is usually satisfying only to an outsider . . . . *In the intensity of the emotional disturbance itself lies the value, the energy which he should have at his disposal in order to remedy the state of reduced adaptation.* . . . In order, therefore, to gain possession of the energy that is in the wrong place, he must . . . . make himself as conscious as possible of the mood he is in, sinking himself in it without reserve and noting down on paper all the fantasies and other associations that come up.[4]

Jung suggested several methods of treating depression based on

---

[3] CW 5, par. 625.

[4] "The Transcendent Function," *The Structure and Dynamics of the Psyche,* CW 8, pars. 166-167 (italics in original).

his clinical experience. For example, he advised against adopting a supportive stance. Discussing a female patient who went into a deep depression every time he went on a vacation, he pointed out that if he sacrificed himself for the patient it would only drive her deeper into her depression. According to Jung, she always survived his absence because something came up in her that lifted the depression.[5]

He also advised against trying to talk depressive patients out of their negative feelings and ideas.

> These negative feelings are so many auto-suggestions which he accepts without argument. Intellectually, he can understand them perfectly and recognize them as untrue, but nevertheless the feelings persist. They cannot be attacked by intellect because they have no intellectual or rational basis.[6]

Summary

Jung recognized depression as a normal accompaniment to personality development and not necessarily pathological. This led him to appreciate the relationship between normal depression and the process of transformation. Depression in such instances is purposive.

In addition, Jung's ego-depletion theory is capable of explaining many symptoms characteristic of depressive disorder. For example, the symbolic association between money and libido can explain the fact that depressed individuals commonly suffer from feelings of impoverishment regardless of their economic circumstances. Similarly, feelings of helplessness and hopelessness are readily associated with the lack of energy available to the depleted ego.

Jung's therapeutic approach is derived from, and theoretically consistent with, his ideas on how the personality functions and how pathology develops. It recognizes the importance of the unconscious in the etiology and treatment of depression. The resolution of a depression, he says, must come ultimately from an understanding of its unconscious meanings. His approach alludes to the necessity of regression and the significance of understanding unresolved infantile

---

[5] *The Visions Seminars*, pp. 53-54.
[6] "The Relations Between the Ego and the Unconscious," *Two Essays on Analytical Psychology*, CW 7, par. 344.

conflicts. Many of Jung's technical ideas, especially those derived from his clinical experience, are consistent with current research. In addition, he developed a creative approach to help those who suffer from depression associated with the transformative process.

Since Jung was primarily interested in transformative depression, he did not fully explore the clinical implications of his concepts. Part II of this chapter will extend Jung's ideas and reformulate them in the light of current research into depressive disorder. All the issues examined revolve around one central theme—the archetypal idea of redemption through submission.

Part II: Redemption Through Submission

Etiology

People suffering from depressive disorder are dominated by sadness and self-reproach. They believe that their negative thoughts and feelings are a correct assessment of themselves, the world they live in and their future existence. In contrast, those who experience normal depression consider their mood to be alien and struggle against it.

Bowlby suggests that normal depression is a mood that is the natural accompaniment of any state in which behavior becomes disorganized, as is likely after a loss.[7] Jung says that depression is the normal consequence of a compensatory encounter with the unconscious. Jung's position is compatible with Bowlby's if it is understood that contact with the unconscious has a disorienting effect on the ego. Depression in such cases has a purpose because a new, healthier adaptation cannot develop without first dismantling the old. A person not subject to depressive disorder can suffer through change and emerge with behavior, thought and feeling reorganized on a new level. There is no permanent damage to self-esteem as a result of the experience. Those who are subject to depressive disorder, however, degenerate. Unless there is professional intervention, they emerge weaker than before, with no new adaptation and with seriously damaged self-esteem.

What factors make some individuals prone to depressive disorder

---

[7] J. Bowlby, *Attachment and Loss,* vol. 3, chapts. 11, 12, 14, 21.

while others react to similar circumstances with a normal or trans-formative depression?

Jung discusses a number of events that can lead to depressive disorder. The loss of energy can come about through avoidance of conscious responsibilities and activities which cause energy to be damned up and flow into the unconscious. At other times Jung attributes depression to rejection and loss. Similarly, Harding says the blocking of libido and consequent regression can be caused by

> some set-back in life . . . disappointment because something one had anticipated has failed to materialize, or a cherished plan has fallen through, or an ego wish has been frustrated. . . . the death of a loved one, the break-up of a marriage, serious illness, failure in business, or the collapse of all one's hopes and ambitions.[8]

A difficulty with the formulations of both Jung and Harding is that there is no inherent reason for any of the stated precipitants to result in a blockage of libido and a depressive illness. Quite the contrary; in many people setbacks result in adaptive behavior. In these cases, rather than a regression of libido characteristic of depression, there is a continuance of the progression of libido. To account for these differences some writers have hypothesized a predisposition to develop depressive illness, which, they suggest, is based on either constitutional factors or events that occurred in a person's childhood, or some combination of the two.[9]

My own clinical experience indicates that one significant factor in the development of depression is a severe loss of love early in life and the development of the idea that some personal evil was responsible. This idea is often strengthened by parental remarks such as "You'll be the death of me," or overt threats of abandonment for misbehavior. Of even more significance, however, is that the loss of love is preceded by an extended experience of feeling loved by one or both parents.

Spitz carried out observations on 123 infants in the nursery of a

---

[8] "The Meaning and Value of Depression," p. 3.

[9] K. Abraham, "Notes on the Psycho-Analytical Investigation and Treatment of Manic-Depressive Insanity and Allied Conditions"; E. Bibring, "The Mechanism of Depression"; D. Abse, "The Depressive Character"; G. Kirschner, "The Depressive Process Examined in View of Creativity."

criminal institution.[10] He noticed that many infants developed symptoms that were remarkably similar to adult melancholia. The one factor which all who developed the depressive syndrome had in common was that the mother had been separated from the child somewhere around the eighth month for approximately three months. In each case depressive symptoms developed. No child whose mother remained with it developed the depressive syndrome. On the other hand, not all children whose mothers were gone became depressed.

In the institution, after separation from the mother, another inmate was assigned to the care of the motherless child. It was discovered that it was more difficult to replace a satisfactory mother than an unsatisfactory one, so that depression was more frequent and more severe in the cases of good mother-child relationships. In bad mother-child relationships not a single severe depression occurred. In essence, the child must first have had love and then lost it in order to become depressed. If the child never had a loving relationship to begin with, depression did not develop.

Spitz' research corroborates my own observations with adult depressives. They all report a period early in life when they felt loved, and a subsequent period when they did not. Their depression seems to be an attempt to regain love, as well as a reaction to its loss. All of the analysands report that their fathers were initially very loving. At some point the fathers suddenly and without explanation withdrew. Two fathers withdrew at early signs of independent behavior in their daughters; one withdrew when his wife developed a psychotic depression accompanied by the delusion that their daughter was stealing the husband. Fathers of two men withdrew into alcoholism at losses having nothing to do with the analysands. In all these cases, however, the children blamed themselves and attempted to redeem the lost love by behaving in a submissive fashion.

The mothers of three women had all suffered their own very severe depressions for most of their lives. These depressions preceded marriage, were exacerbated by childbirth and then continued for an extended duration. The mothers of two men suffered prolonged organic illness when their sons were under four years of age; the moth-

---

10 "Anaclitic Depression: An Inquiry into the Genesis of Psychiatric Conditions in Early Childhood."

ers were probably depressed during this period or at least largely inaccessible.

As a result of the original loving care and the idea that their own evil caused its loss, these depressives developed the belief that if they found the proper form of behavior they could make others become loving again. Thus, while they despair, they are unconsciously hopeful, harboring the idea that the other has not been lost irrevocably, based on the experience that the other once *was* loving. The attendant hope is that the redemption of others will also redeem their own positive feelings about themselves.

Introversion-Extraversion

It was once thought that depressives manifest a lack of interest in the external environment. Jung explained their withdrawal by equating depression with introversion, necessary to compensate a too extraverted orientation. In these terms, depression is a symptom/ symbol pointing to the pressing need to attend to the inner life.

I have found that people who suffer depressive disorders generally live extremely extraverted lives. Because of their particular childhood experiences, they developed extraversion as a defense against the threat of loss that leads to disorganization and then to severe depression. They were usually raised in households where they were forbidden any modes of understanding other than those directed by the parents. Behavior other than submission to the parents' construction of reality led to the threat of loss of love. As a consequence of living in such an atmosphere, these individuals became sensitively attuned to the needs of others.

This leads depression-prone individuals to be afraid of introversion. This is due not only to the fear of discovering something in the unconscious that will set off a depressive cycle, but also because the very process of paying attention to their inner lives may have frightening consequences. Both looking within and the subsequent recognition of their own unique nature are acts of separateness and independence. These are the very qualities depression-prone individuals most fear. They avoid introversion in order to protect themselves from threatened loss of love. At the same time and for the same reason, they develop extraversion to an extreme degree.

Jung's idea that depression is a form of pathological or forced introversion, and the related idea that depression is a compensation for extraversion, leads to several problems. In particular, people in a state of depression do not seem to be introverting on any level. Instead, they seem to be obsessing about delusions concerning their own negativity. This obsession occurs when there is a breakdown in their extraverted attempts to stave off bad feelings about themselves through submission. Are they then in a state of forced introversion, or is this simply another form of submissive extraversion?

A number of authors have suggested that the self-centered ruminations of the depressive are a diversionary defense against the painful feelings of loss that are really the problem.[11] The depressive is avoiding the introverted experience that would entail an exploration of the unconscious and an understanding of the source of sadness. Normally, one may introvert due to some painful experience, become depressed for a time and then ultimately adapt. But this is not what happens to a severely depressed person. Instead, attention is diverted to obsessive negative thoughts. The depressive does this because he or she has learned to deal with loss and pain by first submitting as weak and inferior to a dominant parent figure, and then being saved by that same other.[12]

In such cases, extraversion is an expression of the same psychological force that predisposes some people toward depression; it is a defense against loss of love. Instead of being a form of introversion, the depression is a continuation of the pattern that leads to extreme extraversion. Both are a form of turning away from exploration of the inner life.

Depressive disorder is the end result of a breakdown of the system of which extraversion is one expression. It is a system designed to attain redemption through submission to a powerful figure who is capable of saving a person by imparting love and meaning to life.

---

11 E.J. Sacher, J.M. Mackenzie, W.A. Binstock and J.E. Mack, "Corticosteroid Responses to the Psychotherapy of Reactive Depressions. II. Further Clinical and Physiological Implications," pp. 23-44; J.H. Smith, "Identificatory Styles in Depression and Grief," pp. 259-266.

12 S. Arieti and J. Bemporad, *Severe and Mild Depression*, pp. 129-185.

When this attempt at redemption is experienced as a failure and the earlier primal loss of love is reexperienced, depression ensues. But severely depressed people are dominated by the extraverted orientation even while in the depression. They still focus on the outer world in a continuing attempt to read others' needs more successfully so that they can fulfill these needs and be redeemed.

It is also questionable whether, under these circumstances, the extraversion experienced by the depression-prone individual is a true extraversion. The person's libido is not necessarily following a natural gradient of interest in the other. Instead, the individual has learned to submit to and satisfy the other for the sake of the other's approval and pleasure, not for personal satisfaction or intrinsic interest in the outer world.

From the clinical point of view, those prone to severe depression do need to learn to be more introverted. They must be helped to face the fear of loss and the sense of emptiness they have come to associate with being attuned to their inner lives. Similarly, they need to understand that extraversion is not necessarily a function of their interest in others or their natural adaptation to life; rather, it is a technique used to gain approval at the expense of their own needs. Depressives also need to learn that both their extraversion and their depression are defenses against loss. The goals in the analyses of severe depressives are thus the development of a proper relationship with the demands of the inner life and a true experience of the fascination and joy of the outer.

A sign of improvement in depressives is when their defensively extraverted orientation diminishes and they show incipient signs of introversion. Typically, this manifests as an awareness of personal reactions rather than a concern about how others want them to react. For instance, they begin to pay attention to whether they like another person rather than trying to sense what others require of them.

It is possible to conclude that depression is an extraverted rather than an introverted experience. In the passage quoted earlier from *Symbols of Transformation,* Jung said that depression is due to a regressive looking back and that "regression is also an involuntary introversion." Libido that moves backward—that is, regressively—flows into the unconscious and activates childhood events. Libido that flows inward moves toward subjective awareness. Jung combined the two and said that regression is an involuntary introversion. However, elsewhere Jung wrote that regression can be either introverted or extraverted, "either as a retreat from the outside world (introversion), or as a flight into extravagant experience of the outside world (extraversion)."[13]

Regression and introversion are not synonymous. Thus, on the basis of his own libido theory, Jung's ideas can be reformulated to suggest that a depression can be both extraverted and regressive, which better fits the clinical evidence and accounts for the ego's depleted state, the defensive extraverted orientation of the depressive and the regressively activated infantile conflicts.

Aggression

The excessive and irrational guilt and self-reproach depressed individuals suffer is often induced by parents who threaten to withdraw their love from a nonconforming child. Such threats typically center on the child's self-assertiveness, which the parents experience as hostility. The child learns to associate assertion with being unlovable.

To ensure obedience some parents induce a sense of guilt by telling the child that its behavior is making one of the parents seriously ill. Often the child is made to feel it is intrinsically unlovable because of this aggressiveness, or is pressured to care for a sick, anxious, depressed or hypochondriacal parent. This leads the child to feel responsible for the parent's care, since its aggression was responsible for the illness in the first place.

I worked with a depressed woman who was raised by a depressed mother. At first she had blamed her father's brutality for her mother's depression. With her mother's encouragement, however, the patient developed the idea that she was guilty for not having intervened to stop him beating the mother. She was told that her attempts to assert herself had caused the father to beat the mother.

This woman, an excellent dancer, had fantasies of a career related to dance or movement. However, she avoided attending classes and

---

13 "On Psychic Energy," *The Structure and Dynamics of the Psyche,* CW 8, par. 77.

over-ate to the point of obesity. Analysis indicated that she felt guilty about her ability to do the dance movements effortlessly. In her fantasy, the teacher's correction of the other dancers made them feel inferior. The patient blamed herself for making the other dancers depressed and reproached herself for her imagined aggression toward them. She redeemed herself by not doing her own dance work well and avoided class whenever possible.

From her associations it became clear that the other women represented her mother who, the patient felt, had become more depressed when the patient did well in school or became interested in outside activities. Her mother indicated that she felt threatened at being left to the mercy of her brutal husband. In order to cling, the mother reproached her daughter, making her feel guilty by suggesting that her attempts at self-development were aggressive acts.

Most writers on depression note a similar correlation between depression, especially the melancholic variety, and impounded, or forcibly contained, aggression. Whether this correlation is causative and, if so, how, is subject to controversy.

Some writers see depression as a direct result of impounded aggression. Freud, for instance, developed the idea that the self-reproaches of the depressive were not really directed toward the self at all, but toward some person the depressive loves or feels he or she should love.[14] Much of the symptomatology of depression, Freud concluded, could be seen as a result of internalized aggression actually meant for a love object. He further asserted that the very thing of which depressive individuals accuse themselves is the anger they experience about others.

Arieti, on the other hand, believed that depression is not primarily a defense against aggressive affects such as power, hate or anger.[15] Although these are repressed in depression-prone individuals, and although depressives do express anger against themselves when it is actually felt toward others, depression is not caused by these affects turned against the self. Rather, the repression of these feelings is a consequence of the psychological set-up that causes the depression.

---

[14] S. Freud, *Mourning and Melancholia,* pp. 237-258.
[15] S. Arieti and J. Bemporad, *Severe and Mild Depression,* pp. 176-181.

To be overtly angry toward another or to indicate a will to power is nonsubmissive behavior and leads to anxiety and guilt. As children, depressive people lost love and were accused of being bad when they asserted themselves. Thus, they learned to associate being unlovable with feeling and expressing aggression. They also feel guilty. As a consequence, they try to win back their sense of goodness and lovableness from rejecting parent figures by repressing the aggressive components in their personalities.

The resolution of this controversy is subject to future research, but, regardless of the outcome, any theory that attempts to deal with depression must consider its relation to aggression. One cannot explain the most obvious characteristic of depression—the guilt and reproach directed against the self and, more subtly, against others—without discussing aggression. This is a primary area for the extension of Jung's thought.

My own clinical experience agrees with those who see aggression as impounded owing to depressive dynamics, and only secondarily turned against oneself. A number of analysands report the experience of fathers who were loving to them when they were infants but who suddenly withdrew when their children began to say no or show other signs of self-assertion. They all experienced a depressing loss, then "understood" the loss as due to their self-assertion, and only then tried to repress their aggression in order to redeem themselves.

One woman felt that her depressed mother was too weak to handle aggression. As a child, she felt she would lose what little approval she still got from her mother if she showed her developing self-assertion. So she suppressed her own needs and submitted to her mother's need for a compliant child who, at the same time, was "independent," that is, made no demands on her. The patient remembers learning to control her aggressive feelings by telling herself they were bad and that she was unlovable for having them.

In these examples, aggressive emotions were repressed and the analysands became submissive. Submissiveness was required to receive love and approval from the parents or, at least, to minimize the threat of their loss. It is this original sense of loss, self-blame and need for redemption via submission that cause a person to become depression prone, not the repression of aggression. On the contrary, the repression of aggression is a consequence of the depressive's psychology, not the cause, and in fact depressives repress almost all intense feelings, not only aggression.

The position taken by the therapist on this issue conditions the analytic interventions. Personally, I find that helping depression-prone analysands become conscious of their aggressive feelings is valuable in many ways, but that consciousness of these alone does not cure the pattern. What does help is their understanding that the very conditions that lead to depression-prone psychology also lead to the denial of aggressive affects.

The analysand needs to understand the following process. An aggressive or self-assertive reaction leads to a fear of loss of love and to guilt. This generates the redemptive reaction of submission. The submission is a combination of intrapsychic defense through repression and interpersonal defense via the depressive symptomatology of overt weakness and self-reproach. Self-reproach uses the angry feelings felt toward the other and directs them against the self.

In melancholia, symptomatic aggression, self-reproach and guilt appear with an incapacitating ferocity. Jung recognized the existence of a melancholic depression, and flirted briefly with a somatogenic hypothesis as an explanation when he suggested that melancholia was caused by a constitutional melancholic mood.[16] However, he never elaborated on the subject except to say that melancholia was caused by something other than the pull of unconscious fantasies.

An important issue is the relationship between the intense guilt and self-reproach of melancholia and their relatively milder manifestation in simple depression. This question is related to the larger issue of whether simple depressions and melancholic depressions are independent disorders with distinct etiologies and dynamics, or whether they exist on a continuum, with melancholia as the more extreme form with additional dynamics. The therapeutic approach is partly determined by this issue.

If simple and melancholic depressions exist on a continuum, then one would expect to see a movement between melancholic and simple depression during the course of psychotherapy. If they are com-

---

[16] "On Manic Mood Disorder," *Psychiatric Studies*, CW 1, par. 191.

pletely distinct, this progression would be absent.

A woman came to her analytic session suffering from a recent up-surge of melancholic depression. During a date with her ex-husband she had begun to feel intense inferiority and self-reproach. Analysis revealed that she was only seeing him because of a need to feel liked, not because of her interest in him. In truth, she felt angry at his self-centered, negative behavior. She had not recognized that the negative thoughts and feelings she had about herself were really felt toward him. Consciousness of her hostile feelings caused a change in her depression. The damage to her narcissism caused by her self-re-proaches ceased, indicating that the repressed aggression had turned against her in the form of self-reproach.

At her next session she felt deprived of energy, unable to motivate herself and helpless, though she was free of melancholic self-re-proach. Her residual depression was traced to a conflict over her negative feelings. Recognition of her anger against her ex-husband had aroused an underlying inner conflict with the image of her mother, which centered on the analysand's experience of loss of love and an urge to submit in order to appease the rejecting parent. Although consciousness of her aggressive feelings meant she could no longer use them as a basis for self-reproach, she remained de-pleted by the underlying conflict.

This example, and a number of similar experiences with other analysands, suggests that melancholic depressions do exist on a con-tinuum with simple depressions, compounded by self-reproach be-cause of repressed aggression turned against oneself. Analysis of these cases suggests that the tendency to turn aggression inward is related to parental criticism and aggressive attitudes toward the child. Those who suffer melancholic depressions have experienced this criticism earlier, more continuously and more severely than those who experience simple depression.

Psychotherapy

Jung saw a distinction between depression as a normal process and as a pathology. He did not, however, distinguish normal depression from pathological depression in his therapeutic approach, designed to present the ego with unconscious contents necessary to compensate its one-sided attitude.

Nor did Jung specify whether there were particular psychological issues that had a tendency to cause depression. Instead, he generalized that whatever complex is activated in the unconscious draws libido to it. To discover the unconscious complex that is drawing off the ego's energy and creating the depression, one has to follow the regressed libido into the unconscious. Fantasies are encouraged, as are painting, sculpting and other means of objectification. It is assumed that with the analyst's encouragement the patient will integrate these contents, acquire the libido of which the contents are manifestations, and thereby relieve the depression. Clinical experience indicates, however, that a person suffering a serious depressive disorder will merely produce obsessive negative thoughts and images.

Rather than just encouraging a relationship to the unconscious, it is helpful for analysts to be aware of the particular conflicts and dynamic patterns associated with depressive disorder, and to utilize this knowledge to orient themselves. By understanding the etiology and dynamics of a particular disorder the analyst can choose from the vast amount of unconscious material presented in a session what is most pertinent to the analysand's condition. Otherwise there is a danger of interpreting, or avoiding the interpretation of, unconscious material based on the resistances of the patient or the analyst's own neurotic countertransference.

A therapeutic approach to depression must also take account of how the ego of the depressive reacts to the unconscious. The discovery of unconscious contents often leads to further depression. This is due to the association in the mind of the depressive between individual existence and loss of love. Interpretation by the analyst results in the patient either submitting to the analyst's point of view or uttering depressive comments designed to make the analyst feel helpless.

Failure to distinguish normal from pathological depression can lead to errors deleterious to treatment. The analyst should relate to transformative depression with support and content interpretation. Serious depressive disorders, however, require a different type of treatment. Depressives expect support, love and approval in return for submissive behavior, a pattern established early in childhood.

Transference and countertransference dynamics become critical in such situations. Intense demands are made on the analyst to assume the role of the dominant parental figures in return for submissive behavior. Supporting this reinforces the pathological equation learned in childhood, that depressed behavior elicits loving support. What is necessary, therefore, are transference-countertransference interpretations that bring to consciousness the specific dynamics relating depressive symptomatology to parental love.

Transference and Countertransference Reactions

Transference and countertransference reactions that occur during the analysis of depressed patients differ in many significant ways from those that occur in the analysis of patients with other disorders. In chapter five I discussed the relationship between idealization and depression. Here I will discuss the analyst's reactions to the depressed patient's conflicts over dependence.

Dependence-Independence

Seriously depressed people are very dependent and have severe conflicts about their dependency. They have strong associations, originating from early childhood, to loss of love resulting from independence, on the one hand, and then to the possibility of regaining it by becoming dependent, on the other. Their conflicts usually manifest in the transference in one of two ways: either the analysand is overly dependent, or there is a flight into an extreme, but false, independence.

Those who are overly dependent make intense claims on the analyst. They become demanding, critical and angry if the analyst fails to respond to their helplessness with advice, control or other caretaking actions. They do not consider interpretation to be an adequate expression of care and support. Instead, they feel the analysis is not helping: they are getting worse and are even more depressed. The analyst must *do* something, not just interpret.

The countertransference reactions usually engendered in the analyst are feelings of guilt and incompetence. The analyst wonders if enough is being done and redoubles efforts to make the pithy interpretation that will catalyze a breakthrough and relieve the patient's suffering. Such an interpretation is also rejected, of course, because interpretation is not what the patient wants. The analyst then feels incompetent and inadequate, and eventually becomes angry. Either overtly or covertly, the analyst blames the patient for not letting "good" interpretations have the desired effect. Often the analyst will then suggest that the depression is too severe and must be lifted before interpretive therapy can be effective. A short treatment with antidepressants may be recommended.

A further complication of this countertransference reaction to overt dependency occurs when the analyst identifies with the nourishing aspect of the Great Mother archetype and tries to emotionally care for and support the patient. The analyst thinks that once the patient feels loved, then the analyst's insights will be accepted. Experience demonstrates that this does not work. While there may be short-term improvement, there is no lasting effect on the tendency for depression to recur. The countertransference is seriously compounded in analysts who also identify with the hero or savior archetype.

In such situations the analyst must understand that he or she is experiencing the same feelings as the analysand. The analyst's depressed feelings of loss of love, guilt and incompetence, and simultaneous anger with self and patient, are exactly what the patient feels. The analyst has lost love because he or she does not live up to the patient's demands or reward submission. The analyst feels guilty and incompetent and angrily blames the patient because the analyst depends on the patient's approval in order to get rid of the depressed feelings. This is, of course, a replication in the analyst of the patient's childhood paradigm, and the present dynamic with the parental imagoes in the patient's unconscious.

The analyst must first understand all of this, then persistently point out that the patient feels like an incompetent child who must be taken care of and who has learned that someone will eventually respond if they make themselves helpless enough. When the patient pleads genuine helplessness, the analyst must point out again that this is because self-sufficiency causes the patient to feel unloved, whereas helplessness and dependence have in the past earned some measure of love.

The other type of depression-prone analysand is equally dependent but tenaciously resists becoming attached to the analyst. Such people are only too aware of their extreme dependency feelings. Sometimes they will even admit to them, but they immediately add that they hate these feelings and do not want to give in to them. They will often behave in a manner of exaggerated independence when they are not in a depressive downswing. They always have at least one seriously depressed parent, usually the mother. They understood at an early age that their mothers could not tolerate their dependency needs and withdrew in response. These mothers taught their children to be independent but in a dependent way; that is, the children learned always to act independently, even when they were feeling dependent, so that their mothers would not withdraw. Their independence became a form of submission in return for love.

One patient with a depressed mother was taking care of the domestic needs of the entire family while still a young child. She cooked all the meals and cleaned the house because her mother could not. She felt that by doing all the work she was getting silent approval from her depressed mother. Another woman also remembered becoming independent very early because she realized that her mother withdrew even further into her own depression whenever the patient became dependent. She, too, took over the job of keeping the house in order.

These patients live out this pattern with the analyst. Although they feel dependent early in the analysis, they only show it after they have collapsed completely into a severe depression. Then they hate themselves for being so weak. As soon as they are able, they try to reassert their independent stance. In their transference fantasies they assume that the analyst, like the depressed parent, really requires this of them.

The countertransference reaction toward such analysands is different from that with overtly dependent people. Here, the analyst experiences the longing for dependence that these patients hate in themselves. The analyst tends to talk about the normalcy of depending on others and to explain that it is not necessary to experience self-hate. The analyst's choice of this approach, however, is often based on his or her own unconscious need to feel needed. This behavior protects the analyst from the anxiety that would be aroused if the patient no longer needed the analyst.

This reaction also misses the essential psychological dynamic operating in these patients; that is, they are already behaving in a dependent manner. Their "independent" behavior is entirely submissive to what they fantasize the depressed mother/analyst needs them to be. These patients, in the extraverted way characteristic of depressives, are not attending to their own needs and behaving independently because of their own feelings and perceptions. Instead, they are behaving in the indirectly dependent, submissive way they learned in childhood.

An example of this relationship is that of a depressed couple, where the man held the position of the weak, dependent one. The wife took the position of the strong, independent partner, just as she had with her depressed mother. This woman resented always having to be strong and independent and never being able to satisfy her needy, dependent feelings, but she was afraid that her husband, as her mother before, would become angry and withdraw. In addition, she felt extreme self-hate when she did behave in a dependent way. When she began to understand that her independent behavior with her husband was really a continuation of her submission to and dependence on her depressed mother, she gained some insight into her dependence-independence conflicts.

Theoretical Considerations

The motif of redemption is significant for those who suffer depressive disorders. Depressives try to redeem themselves with those people who threaten to or actually do withdraw love; they also try to redeem themselves with those whom they fantasize will withdraw love. The contemporary experience is symbolic of the more significant primary loss in childhood. The process of redemption through submission is intended to transform the other into a redeemer, from a bad, unloving person into a good and loving one. If the depressed person is successful in this, he or she experiences a mitigation of self-hate, guilt, helplessness and hopelessness.

What is interesting about this process is that it often works, at least temporarily. A significant other can save the depressive from immediate suffering. The depression lifts and the depressive experiences relatively decent feelings about self and the world. The therapist who has managed, through love and support, to help a depressed patient out of depression usually feels quite successful. Unfortunately, the "cure" does not last; the next real or imagined loss sets off another depressive downswing. What is worse, though, is that in submitting to what others think—or what the depressive imagines they think—the depressive suffers loss of soul. Such an individual holds on to a facsimile of love while becoming alienated from a sense of self. This makes one even more vulnerable and dependent on others to give meaning and value to life. This is the bargain a depressive makes.

The redemptive process of the depressive is contrary to the purpose and significance of redemption as understood from the points of view of Christianity, alchemy and fairy tales. Jung points out that in both Christianity and alchemy the redeeming value of the Self is projected: onto Christ in one case and onto the *lapis* in the other.[17]

In Christianity, the work of redemption which brings about the reconciliation of man with God is left to the autonomous divine figure. The alchemist attributes the state of suffering and need for redemption to the divine soul that is imprisoned in matter. The work of redemption, the opus, is carried out by the alchemist whose personal salvation becomes an incidental effect of freeing the *anima mundi*. In fairy tales suffering is attributed to curses and bewitchment. Von Franz says that bewitchment is psychologically analogous to a neurosis that comes from a one-sided ego attitude.[18] Redemption here is a function of an instinctive "right" response. This is only possible via a connection to the wholeness of a situation through the Self.

In all of these circumstances the goal of the redemptive work is the improvement of a relationship with the Self. But for the depressive, the significance of redemption comes not from connection with the Self, but from connection with parents or projected parental imagoes. The reestablishment of the relationship to the parental figures is the

---

[17] *Psychology and Alchemy*, CW 12, pars. 414-424.
[18] *Redemption Motifs in Fairy Tales*, p. 7.

goal of the work; the relationship to the Self is sacrificed in the process. Why this happens introduces a question raised earlier: Why do some people react to contact with the unconscious with an adaptive depression while others react with a depressive disorder?

In the course of its growth, the ego must establish an adequate relationship between the outer environment and the unconscious. Ego development can be seen as a series of disorganizations resulting from compensatory experiences that are accompanied by normal depression. This leads to subsequent integration of the ego on a more psychologically adapted level. The newly reorganized ego represents a greater approximation to the Self. Depressions associated with this process are adaptive and creative.

While the ego as a personal identity structure tends toward conservatism, as a psychological structure with a teleological orientation it is meant to transform. Transformation leads to actualization of the Self in the phenomenal world. Jung called this process of directional change the individuation process.

A significant part of this process is the apprehension and surrender of the ego to the demands of the Self. The ego must sacrifice its environmentally conditioned values and behaviors and, whenever possible, adopt the instinctive response that represents the total personality. A proper relationship to the hero archetype is important at this juncture. If the hero is thought of not as a symbol of the ego, but, as von Franz suggests, as the ego-building function of the Self, then the hero presents the ego with the instinctively right response to a situation based on the Self's perception.[19] To follow through with the right response is what redeems the ego from its curse in fairy tales. The ego is redeemed from its limited, one-sided state by becoming a closer approximation of the Self. It becomes more individuated.

This, however, is not what happens to people with depressive disorders. Rather than surrendering to the inner demands of the Self, the depressive submits to the personal demands of the parental imagoes. This happens because the ego's identity is in no way related to the Self. When the ego-building function of the Self, as expressed

---

[19] Ibid., p. 19.

through the hero archetype, becomes active, depression-prone individuals suffer the disorder. The activity of the Self instantly and unconsciously brings up the childhood paradigm. To receive love the child had to live out the ideals of the parents, reflecting their glory, not that of the Self. Self-assertion, which springs from a child's innate sense of the right response to a situation, was met by the withdrawal of a "loving" father or a depressed mother. The loss of love was followed by self-blame and other depressive symptomatology encouraged by the parents. Submission to parental demands brought saving relief. Over time, the child learned that self-awareness and attention to the Self brought depression, while extraversion that gratified the needs of others prevented it. As a consequence the ego did not grow independently but was modeled after the expectations of the parents and the culture..

Submission to environmental demands is a necessary stage in all ego development and leads to the ability to deal adequately with the collective. By itself, however, it leads to the sterile conformity of "good" children. What is missing in them is the ability to say no. Even when, because of practical considerations, a person must deny the Self, it is important not only to be able to bear the tension of consciously knowing that a true need has been denied, but also to be able to feel sadness and loss. There is far less inner disharmony under these circumstances, for the Self has at least been acknowledged.

One of the primary therapeutic tasks is to help the patient realize that he or she tries to avoid the depression by sacrificing the relationship to the Self. The symbol the depressive lives under, submission to a greater force in order to redeem love, is a religious motif. It is played out on the personal level by the ego's submission to the initial carriers of the projected Self, namely the parental imagoes. The depressive feels temporarily relieved because this does have a redeeming effect. Depression lurks, though, because a person's sense of self-worth, which must be founded on a relationship to the Self, has been sacrificed. In return for a facsimile of parental love, the person has sacrificed Self-love.

Patients with depressive disorders understand their situation differently. They see the necessity for submission, but live it out on the level of a symptom. They must learn to listen to the Self and surrender to their own inner responses. They must give up the symptom, the desperate attempt to win love from the parents in return for submission, and embrace the symbol, the Self. True redemption comes from surrender to the Self, not submission to the parents.

One woman who had suffered a life-long depression was just beginning to be able to experience this distinction, when she decided that she should leave analysis. She felt that the work was in her best interest and meant a great deal to her. She lived a very isolated life and part of her growth had been a commitment to her interpersonal development, strongly affected by the analytic relationship. But she had severe financial difficulties, and after long consideration decided she would have to sacrifice analysis.

Despite the impending loss, she did not have a depressive reaction. Instead, she suffered normal feelings of loss and sadness. This was an important psychological achievement.

In her last session before terminating, she had the spontaneous feeling that, despite her very real economic hardship, she really ought to remain in the analysis. She immediately felt depressed. At first, this reaction was confusing. Depression could be expected when she was preparing to leave, not when she decided to stay.

During our discussion, the following intrapsychic dynamic emerged. At the moment she had the spontaneous response to stay in analysis, she had a feeling of its rightness. It came from a good inner source. This was immediately followed by the image of an angry parental figure who was furious at her for surrendering.

"Surrendering to whom?" I asked.

"To my need for personal development," she replied. "This image is furious because rather than surrendering to it, I am surrendering to myself. That is what I am depressed about. Doing what is right for me is depressing."

Epilogue

What leads to positive change in the patient's condition? This is a critical question for psychotherapy. The generally accepted model is that making the unconscious conscious via interpretation results in the withdrawal of infantile and archetypal projections. This allows for the development of psychic balance and new, healthier adaptations.

When a correct interpretation is made, two things occur. Cognitively, patients gain insight into how their psyche operates. Theoretically, this information causes them to feel and behave differently.

Secondly, the analyst has paid very careful attention, and has been interested enough in them to have observed something they were not aware of. The analyst expresses his or her observations in a nonjudgmental and supportive manner. Thus, a particular kind of relating occurs around the interpretation.

Is it the new information that leads to therapeutic effects? Or is it the particular qualities of the therapeutic relationship which are the critical factors?

In addition to the positive effects of interpretation, Jung recognized that the analyst's psyche effects the progress of the patient's treatment.[1] Whether or not this effect is positive naturally depends on the analyst's psychological development, especially in areas where the patient too has conflicts. A psychologically healthy analyst can contribute greatly to the patient's ability to overcome an inferior adaptation. However, if the analyst has an infantile adaptation, the patient's infantile approach to life will be confirmed.

Jung also stressed both the need for healthy relationships to lead the patient out of the family neurosis and the value the patient derived from establishing such a relationship with the analyst.[2] These observations have been supported by clinical research, which indicates that

---

[1] "Some Crucial Points in Psychoanalysis (Jung-Loÿ Correspondence)," *Freud and Psychoanalysis,* CW 4, pars. 661-663.

[2] "The Therapeutic Value of Abreaction," *The Practice of Psychotherapy,* CW 16, pars. 283-286.

effective therapists, regardless of their source of training, operate similarly; they establish an accepting, understanding relationship with their patients.[3]

While therapists tend to attribute the results of successful therapy to their technical skills and insight into unconscious dynamics, patients give precedence to relational factors.[4] Thus, regardless of the rationale behind analytic interpretations, it is the fact of the interpretations being made, combined with the analyst's personality and the "holding quality" of the relationship, that leads the patient to sense an improvement.

But what causes the patient to feel well held? Certainly, except in the most withdrawn and isolated cases, friends and family provide the person with some caring reactions. But accurate interpretive comments by the analyst provide a unique kind of caring, based on understanding. Naturally, the analyst's insightful comments must combine with a therapeutic relationship that differs significantly from painful past relationships, despite the patient's conscious and unconscious compulsion to recreate them with the analyst .

It is through awareness of the transference and countertransference dynamics that the analyst knows when and how the patient's past relationships live in the present. Countertransference reactions help the analyst to understand the patient's expectations and fears. The analyst feels the desire to behave toward the patient as significant others in the patient's past have done; or, conversely, the analyst experiences feelings as the patient did in the past, while the patient identifies with those who inspire these reactions.

Helpful analytic interpretations promote insight and allow the patient the experience of being empathically understood. Just when the patient expects to experience the negative relationship once again, the analyst does something else. Slowly, the patient incorporates an understanding of his or her own psyche and a new set of assumptions about life is established.

---

[3] F. Fiedler, "A Comparison of Therapeutic Relationships in Psychoanalytic, Non-directive and Adlerian Therapy," pp. 436-445.

[4] R.W. Heine, "A Comparison of Patient's Reports on Psychotherapeutic Experience with Psychoanalytic, Non-directive and Adlerian Therapists," pp. 16-23.

Bibliography

Abraham, K. "Notes on the Psycho-Analytical Investigation and Treatment of Manic-Depressive Insanity and Allied Conditions," 1911. In *Psychodynamic Understanding of Depression*, ed. W. Gaylin. New York: Aronson, 1983.

Abse, D. "The Depressive Character." In *Depressive States and Their Treatment*, ed. V. Volkan. New Jersey: Aronson, 1985.

Adler, G. *The Living Symbol*. New York: Pantheon, 1961.

Arieti, S. and Bemporad, J. *Severe and Mild Depression*. New York: Basic Books, 1978.

Bandura, A., and Walters, R. H. *Adolescent Aggression: A Study of the Influence of Child-Rearing Practices and Family Interrelationships*. New York: Ronald Press, 1959.

Barry, W. A. "Marriage Research and Conflict: An Integrative Review." *Psychological Bulletin*, vol. 73 (1970).

Benderly, B. *The Myth of Two Minds: What Gender Means and Doesn't Mean*. New York: Doubleday, 1987.

Bibring, E. "The Mechanisms of Depression." In *Affective Disorders*, ed. P. Greenacre. New York: International University Press, 1953.

Biller, H. B. *Paternal Deprivation*, Lexington, Mass.: Heath, 1974.

Biller, H. B., and Meredith, D. L. *Father Power*. New York: David McKay, 1974.

Bowlby, J. *Attachment and Loss*, vol. 3. New York: Basic Books, 1980.

Brome, V. *Jung: Man and Myth*. New York: Antheum, 1978.

Bronfenbrenner, U. "The Study of Identification Through Interpersonal Perception." In *Person Perception and Interpersonal Behavior*, ed. R. Tagiuri and L. Petrullo. Stanford: Stanford University Press, 1958.

Bronson, W. C. "Dimensions of Ego and Infantile Identification." *Journal of Personality*, vol. 27 (1959).

Burton, R. "Cross-Sex Identity in Barbados." *Developmental Psychology*, vol. 6 (1972).

Carotenuto, A. *A Secret Symmetry: Sabina Spielrein Between Jung and Freud*. Trans. Arno Pomerans, John Shepley, Krishna Winston. New York: Pantheon, 1982.

147

Edinger, E. *Ego and Archetype.* Baltimore: Penguin Books, 1973.

Edinger, E. *The Creation of Consciousness: Jung's Myth for Modern Man.* Toronto: Inner City Books, 1984.

Eliade, M. *Rites and Symbols of Initiation.* New York: Harper and Row, 1958.

Fiedler, F. "A Comparison of Therapeutic Relationships in Psychoanalytic, Non-directive and Adlerian Therapy." *Journal of Consulting Psychology,* vol. 14 (1950).

Fordham, M. "Analytical Psychology and Countertransference." In *Countertransference,* ed. L. Epstein and H. Feiner. New York: Aronson, 1979.

Freud, S. *Mourning and Melancholia.* Standard Edition, vol. 14. London: Hogarth Press, 1961.

Gall, M. D. "The Relationship Between Masculinity-Femininity and Manifest Anxiety." *Journal of Clinical Psychology,* vol. 25 (1969).

Goodenough, E. W. "Interest in Persons as an Aspect of Sex Differences in the Early Years." *Genetic Psychology Monographs,* vol. 55 (1957).

Groesbeck, C. Jess. "The Archetypal Image of the Wounded Healer." *Journal of Analytical Psychology,* vol. 20, no. 2 (1975).

Guggenbühl-Craig, A. *Power in the Helping Professions.* New York: Spring Publications, 1971.

Harding, M. Esther. "The Meaning and Value of Depression." New York: Analytical Psychology Club of New York, 1970.

Hartford, T. C., Willis, C. H. and Deabler, H. L. "Personality Correlates of Masculinity-Femininity." *Psychological Reports,* vol. 21 (1967).

Heimann, P. "On Countertransference." *International Journal of Psycho-Analysis,* vol. 31, no. 1 (1950).

Heine, R.W. "A Comparison of Patient's Reports on Psychotherapeutic Experience with Psychoanalytic, Non-directive and Adlerian Therapists." *American Journal of Psychotherapy,* vol. 7 (1953).

Hetherington, E. M. "A Developmental Study of the Effects of Sex of the Dominant Parent on Sex-Role Preference, Identification, and Imitation in Children." *Journal of Personality and Social Psychology,* vol. 2 (1965).

Hetherington, E. M., Cox, M., and Cox, R. "Family Interaction and the Social, Emotional and Cognitive Development of Children Following Divorce." Paper presented at the Johnson and Johnson Conference on the Family, Washington, DC, May 1978.

Jacoby, M. *The Analytic Encounter: Transference and Human Relationship.* Toronto: Inner City Books, 1984.

Jung, C.G. *The Collected Works* (Bollingen Series XX). 20 vols. Trans. R.F.C. Hull. Ed. H. Read, M. Fordham, G. Adler, Wm. McGuire. Princeton: Princeton University Press, 1953-1979.

_____. *The Visions Seminars: Notes of the Seminars, 1930-1934.* Zurich: Spring Publications, 1976.

Kalsched, D. "Narcissism and the Search for Interiority." *Quadrant,* vol. 13, no. 2 (1980).

Kernberg, O. *Borderline Conditions and Pathological Narcissism.* New York: Aronson, 1975.

Kirschner, G. "The Depressive Process Examined in Terms of Creativity." In *Depressive States and Their Treatment,* ed. V. Volkan. New Jersey: Aronson, 1985.

Klein, M. "Some Theoretical Conclusions Regarding the Emotional Life of the Infant." In *Envy and Gratitude and Other Works: 1946-1963.* London: Hogarth Press, 1975.

Kohut, H. *Restoration of the Self.* New York: International University Press, 1977.

Langs, R. *The Therapeutic Interaction: A Synthesis.* New York: Aronson, 1977.

Lynn, D. B., and Sawrey, W. L. "The Effects of Father-Absence on Norwegian Boys and Girls." *Journal of Abnormal and Social Psychology,* vol. 59 (1959).

Maccoby, E. E. "Sex Differences in Intellectual Functioning." In *The Development of Sex Differences,* ed. E. E. Maccoby. Stanford: Stanford University Press, 1966.

Mahler, M., Pine, F., and Bergman, A. *The Psychological Birth of The Human Infant.* New York. Basic Books,1976.

Masterson, J. *The Narcissistic and Borderline Disorders.* New York: Brunner/Mazel, 1981.

Mead, M. *Male and Female: A Study of the Sexes in a Changing World.* New York: Dell, 1949.

Meier, C.A. *Ancient Incubation and Modern Psychotherapy.* Trans. Monica Curtis. Evanston, IL: Northwestern University Press, 1967.

Miller, S. *Men and Friendship.* San Leandro, CA: Gateway, 1983.

Money, J., & Ehrhardt, A. A. "Prenatal Hormonal Exposure: Possible Effects on Behavior in Man." In *Endocrinology and Human Behavior,* ed. R. P. Micheal. London: Oxford University Press, 1968.

Monick, E. *Phallos: Sacred Image of the Masculine.* Toronto: Inner City Books, 1987.

Mussen, P. H. "Some Antecedents and Consequents of Masculine Sex-Typing in Adolescent Boys." *Psychological Monographs,* vol. 75 (1961).

Mussen, P. H. "Long-Term Consequents of Masculinity of Interests in Adolescence." *Journal of Consulting Psychology,* vol. 26 (1962).

Neumann, E. *The Origins and History of Consciousness* (Bollingen Series XLII). Princeton: Princeton University Press, 1971.

Parsons, T., and Bales, R.F. *Family, Socialization, and Interaction Process.* Glencoe, IL.: Free Press, 1955.

Person, E. "The Omni-Available Woman and Lesbian Sex: Two Fantasy Themes and Their Relationship to the Male Developmental Experience." In *The Psychology of Men,* ed. G. I. Fogel, F. M. Lane and R. S. Liebert. New York: Basic Books, 1986.

Racker, H. *Transference and Countertransference.* London: Hogarth, 1968.

Reich, A. "On Countertransference." *International Journal of Psycho-Analysis,* vol. 32 (1951).

Sacher, E.J., Mackenzie, J.M., Binstock, W.A., and Mack, J.E. "Corticosteroid Responses to the Psychotherapy of Reactive Depressions. II. Further Clinical and Physiological Implications." *Psychosomatic Medicine,* vol. 30 (1968).

Satinover, J. "The Mirror of Doctor Faustus: The Decline of Art in the Pursuit of Eternal Adolescense." *Quadrant,* vol. 17, no. 1 (1984).

Schwartz-Salant, N. *Narcissism and Character Transformation: The Psychology of Narcissistic Character Disorders.* Toronto: Inner City Books, 1982.

Searles, H.F. "The Patient as Therapist to His Analyst." In *Tactics and Technique in Psychoanalytic Therapy, Vol. II: Transference-Countertransference,* ed. P. Giovacchini. New York: Aronson, 1975.

Sears, P. S. "Child Rearing Factors Related to Playing of Sex-Typed Roles." *American Psychologist,* vol. 8 (1953).

Smith, J.H. "Identificatory Styles in Depression and Grief." *International Journal of Psycho-Analysis,* vol. 52 (1971).

Spitz, R. "Anaclitic Depression: An Inquiry into the Genesis of Psychiatric Conditions in Early Childhood." In *Psychodynamic Understanding of Depression,* ed. W. Gaylin. New York, Aronson, 1983.

Spotnitz, H. *Psychotherapy of Preoedipal Conditions.* New York: Aronson, 1976.

Stern, P. *C.G. Jung: The Haunted Prophet.* New York: Braziller, 1976.

Stein, M. "Power, Shamanism, and Maieutics in the Countertransference." *Chiron,* 1984.

Storr, A. "Review of *A Secret Symmetry: Sabina Spielrein Between Jung and Freud.*" *New York Times Book Review,* May 16, 1982.

Ulanov, A. and Ulanov, B. *Cinderella and Her Sisters: The Envied and the Envying.* Philadelphia: The Westminster Press, 1983.

————. *The Witch and the Clown: Two Archetypes of Human Sexuality.* Wilmette, IL: Chiron, 1987.

Von Franz, M.L. *Redemption Motifs in Fairy Tales.* Toronto: Inner City Books, 1980.

Wehr, G. *Jung: A Biography.* Boston: Shambhala, 1987.

Woodman, M. *The Ravaged Bridegroom: Masculinity in Women.* Toronto: Inner City Books, 1990.

————. "Transference and Countertransference in Analysis Dealing with Eating Disorders." *Chiron,* 1984.

Wyly, J. *The Phallic Quest: Priapus and Masculine Inflation.* Toronto: Inner City Books, 1989.

Index

Studies in Jungian Psychology
by Jungian Analysts

Sewn Paperbacks

Prices and payment in U.S. dollars (except for Canadian orders)

1. The Secret Raven: Conflict and Transformation.
Daryl Sharp (Toronto). ISBN 0-919123-00-7. 128 pp. $14
A practical study of *puer* psychology, including dream interpretation and material on
midlife crisis, the provisional life, the mother complex, anima and shadow. Illustrated.

2. The Psychological Meaning of Redemption Motifs in Fairytales.
Marie-Louise von Franz (Zurich). ISBN 0-919123-01-5. 128 pp. $14
Unique approach to understanding typical dream motifs (bathing, clothes, animals, etc.).

3. On Divination and Synchronicity: The Psychology of Meaningful Chance.
Marie-Louise von Franz (Zurich). ISBN 0-919123-02-3. 128 pp. $14
Penetrating study of irrational methods of divining fate (I Ching, astrology, palmistry, Tarot
cards, etc.), contrasting Western ideas with those of so-called primitives. Illustrated.

4. The Owl Was a Baker's Daughter: Obesity, Anorexia and the Repressed
Feminine. Marion Woodman (Toronto). ISBN 0-919123-03-1. 144 pp. $15
A modern classic, with particular attention to the body as mirror of the psyche in weight
disturbances and eating disorders. Based on case studies, dreams and mythology. Illus.

5. Alchemy: An Introduction to the Symbolism and the Psychology.
Marie-Louise von Franz (Zurich). ISBN 0-919123-04-X. 288 pp. $18
Detailed guide to what the alchemists were really looking for: emotional wholeness. Inval-
uable for interpreting images and motifs in modern dreams and drawings. **84 illustrations.**

6. Descent to the Goddess: A Way of Initiation for Women.
Sylvia Brinton Perera (New York). ISBN 0-919123-05-8. 112 pp. $14
A timely and provocative study of the need for an inner, female authority in a masculine-
oriented society. Rich in insights from mythology and the author's analytic practice.

7. The Psyche as Sacrament: C.G. Jung and Paul Tillich.
John P. Dourley (Ottawa). ISBN 0-919123-06-6. 128 pp. $14
Comparative study from a dual perspective (author is Catholic priest and Jungian analyst),
exploring the psychological meaning of religion, God, Christ, the spirit, the Trinity, etc.

8. Border Crossings: Carlos Castaneda's Path of Knowledge.
Donald Lee Williams (Boulder). ISBN 0-919123-07-4. 160 pp. $15
The first thorough psychological examination of the Don Juan novels, bringing Castaneda's
spiritual journey down to earth. Special attention to the psychology of the feminine.

9. Narcissism and Character Transformation. The Psychology of Narcissistic
Character Disorders. ISBN 0-919123-08-2. 192 pp. $16
Nathan Schwartz-Salant (New York).
A comprehensive study of narcissistic character disorders, drawing upon a variety of
analytic points of view (Jung, Freud, Kohut, Klein, etc.). Theory and clinical material. Illus.

10. Rape and Ritual: A Psychological Study.
Bradley A. Te Paske (Minneapolis). ISBN 0-919123-09-0. 160 pp. $15
Incisive combination of theory, clinical material and mythology. Illustrated.

11. Alcoholism and Women: The Background and the Psychology.
Jan Bauer (Montreal). ISBN 0-919123-10-4. 144 pp. $15
Sociology, case material, dream analysis and archetypal patterns from mythology.

12. Addiction to Perfection: The Still Unravished Bride.
Marion Woodman (Toronto). ISBN 0-919123-11-2. 208 pp. $17
A powerful and authoritative look at the psychology of modern women. Examines dreams,
mythology, food rituals, body imagery, sexuality and creativity. A continuing best-seller
since its original publication in 1982. Illustrated.

30. Touching: Body Therapy and Depth Psychology.
Deldon Anne McNeely (Lynchburg, VA). ISBN 0-919123-29-5. 128 pp. $14
Illustrates how these two disciplines, both concerned with restoring life to an ailing human psyche, may be integrated in theory and practice. Focus on the healing power of touch.

31. Personality Types: Jung's Model of Typology.
Daryl Sharp (Toronto). ISBN 0-919123-30-9. 128 pp. $14
Detailed explanation of Jung's model (basis for the widely-used Myers-Briggs Type Indicator), showing its implications for individual development and for relationships. Illus.

32. The Sacred Prostitute: Eternal Aspect of the Feminine.
Nancy Qualls-Corbett (Birmingham). ISBN 0-919123-31-7. 176 pp. $16
Shows how our vitality and capacity for joy depend on rediscovering the ancient connection between spirituality and passionate love. Illustrated. (Foreword by Marion Woodman.)

33. When the Spirits Come Back.
Janet O. Dallett (Seal Harbor, WA). ISBN 0-919123-32-5. 160 pp. $15
An analyst examines herself, her profession and the limitations of prevailing attitudes toward mental disturbance. Interweaving her own story with descriptions of those who come to her for help, she details her rediscovery of the integrity of the healing process.

34. The Mother: Archetypal Image in Fairy Tales.
Sibylle Birkhäuser-Oeri (Zurich). ISBN 0-919123-33-3. 176 pp. $16
Compares processes in the unconscious with common images and motifs in folk-lore. Illustrates how positive and negative mother complexes affect us all, with examples from many well-known fairy tales and daily life. (Edited by Marie-Louise von Franz.)

35. The Survival Papers: Anatomy of a Midlife Crisis.
Daryl Sharp (Toronto). ISBN 0-919123-34-1. 160 pp. $15
Jung's major concepts—persona, shadow, anima and animus, complexes, projection, typology, active imagination, individuation, etc.—are dramatically presented in the immediate context of an analysand's process. And the analyst's.

36. The Cassandra Complex: Living with Disbelief.
Laurie Layton Schapira (New York). ISBN 0-919123-35-X. 160 pp. $15
Shows how unconscious, prophetic sensibilities can be transformed from a burden into a valuable source of conscious understanding. Includes clinical material and an examination of the role of powerfully intuitive, medial women through history. Illustrated.

37. Dear Gladys: The Survival Papers, Book 2.
Daryl Sharp (Toronto). ISBN 0-919123-36-8. 144 pp. $15
An entertaining and instructive continuation of the story begun in *The Survival Papers* (title 35). Part textbook, part novel, part personal exposition.

38. The Phallic Quest: Priapus and Masculine Inflation.
James Wyly (Chicago). ISBN 0-919123-37-6. 128 pp. $14
Case studies, including dreams, showing ways in which one may recognize a split-off priapic complex. Priapus is seen as an apt metaphor for patriarchal inflation.

39. Acrobats of the Gods: Dance and Transformation.
Joan Dexter Blackmer (Concord, MA/Wilmot, NH). ISBN 0-919123-38-4. 128 pp. $14
What is physical consciousness and how is it achieved? What is the connection between psyche and matter? A timely reminder that without the body there can be no soul.

40. Eros and Pathos: Shades of Love and Suffering.
Aldo Carotenuto (Rome). ISBN 0-919123-39-2. 160 pp. $15
Why do we fear love? Why do we hurt those close to us? Is there a connection between love, suffering and creativity? There is treasure in the darkness of love and pain.

Prices and payment (check or money order) in $U.S. (in Canada, $Cdn)

Add Postage/Handling: 1-2 books, $2; 3-4 books, $4; 5-8 books, $7

INNER CITY BOOKS
Box 1271, Station Q, Toronto, Canada M4T 2P4